José Eduardo de Siqueira

Education in Bioethics

José Eduardo de Siqueira

Education in Bioethics

ScienciaScripts

Imprint

Any brand names and product names mentioned in this book are subject to trademark, brand or patent protection and are trademarks or registered trademarks of their respective holders. The use of brand names, product names, common names, trade names, product descriptions etc. even without a particular marking in this work is in no way to be construed to mean that such names may be regarded as unrestricted in respect of trademark and brand protection legislation and could thus be used by anyone.

Cover image: www.ingimage.com

This book is a translation from the original published under ISBN 978-613-9-62183-5.

Publisher:
Sciencia Scripts
is a trademark of
Dodo Books Indian Ocean Ltd. and OmniScriptum S.R.L publishing group

120 High Road, East Finchley, London, N2 9ED, United Kingdom
Str. Armeneasca 28/1, office 1, Chisinau MD-2012, Republic of Moldova, Europe
Printed at: see last page
ISBN: 978-620-7-27448-2

Bioethics education

Jose Eduardo de Siqueira[*]

PREFACE:

This fascicle brings together two book chapters on Clinical Bioethics published in 2008 and 2016 respectively, the first by Editora Gaia of Sao Paulo and the second by the Federal Council of Medicine, on the occasion of the XI Brazilian Congress of Bioethics, III Brazilian Congress of Clinical Bioethics and III International Conference on Teaching Ethics, held in September 2015 in the Federal District. We participated as organizers of both works. The publications were very well received by university professors in the health area, which showed us the great academic interest in the subject. Bioethics is a new area of knowledge that has been incorporated into the curriculum of medical courses to meet a recommendation from the Ministry of Education to train professionals with greater social commitment and the ability to maintain a respectful dialog with patients who are users of the Unified Health System.

We welcome the current initiative by Novas Edigoes Academicas, which aims to disseminate bioethics to a wider audience than just academics.

Jose Eduardo de Siqueira, May 2018

---

[*] Jose Eduardo de Siqueira : PhD in Medicine from the State University of Londrina (UEL), Master's Degree in Bioethicsfrom the University of Chile, Full Professor of Medicine at the Pontifical Catholic University of Paraná (PUCPR), Professor of Fundamentals of Bioethics and Clinical Bioethics in the Postgraduate Program in Bioethics at PUCPR, Full Member of the Board of the International Association of Bioethics (IAB) (2009-2013), President of the Brazilian Society of Bioethics (SBB) (2005-2007), Full Member of the Paraná Academy of Medicine.

1 THE END OF MEDICAL PATERNALISM

Bernard Lown, a disciple of Samuel Levine, one of the most prominent cardiologists of the 20th century, argued, based on the solid experience of more than 40 years of professional practice, that doctors had unlearned the art of healing. In fact, medicine has never advanced so much in the diagnosis and treatment of the most varied diseases as in the last century, but never has the sick human being felt so distant from the doctor's attention. In his book *"The Lost Art of Healing"*, Lown deplores the exaggerated emphasis that medical schools place on training professionals to be, in his words, "chief scientific officers and managers of complex biotechnologies", disregarding the genuine art of being a doctor. He pointed out that true "medical wisdom" is the ability to understand a clinical problem not in terms of an organ, but in terms of the whole human being and, in the end, he denounced: *"(...) the doctor is sought with the right person.) "we seek the doctor with whom we feel at ease when we describe our complaints, without fear of being subjected to numerous procedures; the doctor for whom the patient is never a statistic (...) but, above all, a fellow human being whose concern for the patient is enlivened by the joy of serving (...)"* (LOWN, B.1997).). Equivocally, the thesis that every ailment afflicting the patient can be identified by technology is still held. We have made extraordinary progress in our knowledge of diseases, forgetting about the sick human being and starting to treat diseases of people rather than people who happen to be ill. Young students are taught to operate equipment and to read countless biological variables, but they are not taught to recognize the human being as a biopsychosocial and spiritual unit.

Rozenman recounted the "via crucis" of an elderly patient undergoing coronary artery bypass grafting who, in the late post-operative period, began to suffer from fever and anemia. Admitted to a renowned US hospital, he was examined by a team of competent specialists and underwent numerous semiology procedures, including upper gastrointestinal endoscopy, colonoscopy and computed tomography of the spine followed by spinal biopsy. Diagnostic suspicions ranged from multiple myeloma to cancer with metastasis in the spine, until an adequate physical examination identified the presence of an important systolic murmur in the mitral focus and the diagnosis of infective endocarditis was finally established and confirmed by blood culture identifying *Staphylococcus epidermidis* as the etiologic agent. The author draws attention to the tortuous route used to establish the definitive diagnosis, showing that the countless specialists summoned to give their opinion on the disease did so after lengthy and thorough investigation "within their specific areas of knowledge", disregarding the most basic medical teaching that recognizes the human body as a complex unit made up of organs and systems that interact in a continuous and uninterrupted way. There is not even one stimulus coming from the external environment that is not perceived by the Central Nervous System, immediately passed on to all the other organ systems and which results in the expression of some human feeling (ROZENMAN, Y., 1997).

The search for the "Great Health" imagined by Sfez in the globalized utopia of the 21st century seems to point to a society structured under the rules of *the* most extreme scientific objectivity where *"no one will mourn the death of the doctor, nor that of destiny, nor even that of the soul, another old age, replaced by a collective entity"*. (SFEZ,L., 1996.) Faced with the growing substitution of clinical reasoning for the information provided by sophisticated equipment in today's biomedical technology, it is worth asking whether, at some point, health professionals will not be dispensable for making clinical decisions. There are already programs available on countless virtual platforms that allow interaction between observer and machine, in such a way as to make it possible to carry out diagnoses accompanied by therapeutic approaches, which now do not require medical consultation. If scientific knowledge is entirely stored in machines, wouldn't it be enough for users to access these virtual sources to obtain solutions to their health problems? Is it possible to disregard the incessant search for medical information on the now famous Dr. Google? However, every health professional knows from personal experience that any illness is unlikely to manifest itself exclusively in the organic or psychic, social or family spheres, because they recognize that it will always be both organic and psychic, social and family, a condition that can never be detected by a machine equipped with artificial intelligence. What's more, when a patient seeks medical attention, they are invariably looking for care that is not limited to simply getting rid of a circumstantial ailment. The doctor-patient relationship will never cease to be an intersubjective exercise experienced by two people - health professional and patient - which will only be effective if it is conducted with acceptance, active listening, respectful dialog and hope for a cure for the sufferer.

The symptoms that bring a patient to a consultation always carry a significant amount of mystery. What's behind that persistent headache or that young banker's chest pain? If the blood pressure seen on physical examination is 150 x 100, is that enough to diagnose hypertension? Is prescribing a hypotensive drug with the aim of correcting the abnormal pressure level observed enough to consider the treatment to have been carried out? Symptoms are messages that need to be decoded. The reductionist model enshrined in Cartesian medicine has made real the unlikely linearity between physical symptoms, abnormal blood pressure levels and hypertensive disease. A good anamnesis can reveal that the real cause of headache and hypertension lies in the stressful work environment, so prescribing hypotensives is a maleficent and inappropriate practice. The correct remedy would be to welcome the young person and, through active listening, understand them as a person made vulnerable by the stressful work environment. It would be unreasonable, however, to subject him to an extensive and costly investigation in search of the identification of an organic pathology that justifies the presence of hypertension. This is a mute art that consists of recognizing an illness only through physical signs. The doctor who does this undoubtedly deserves to be replaced by Dr. Google. This model of medicine is far removed from that proposed by Gaillard for the actions of health professionals in the 21st century. The author points to six necessary stages to characterize them. The first would be the welcome, followed by anamnesis and physical examination. The last three stages are diagnosis, prescription and separation. The biggest obstacle to fulfilling these stages, apart from Cartesian training, comes through clearly in the indignant statements made by the French doctors heard by the researcher: "Faced with the low amount of our fees, do you really think we can find time for all these things?" (GAILLARD, J.R.,1995).

Unfortunately, medical care practiced today points to a cruel reality that can be summed up as follows: attend to the patient in the shortest possible time, prescribe any drug and as soon as possible get rid of this uncomfortable and underpaid commitment. Professional and patient, physically so close and affectively so distant, hardly look at each other or touch each other. In fact, they don't even respect each other. In this way, the most perverse model of healthcare is practiced: blind and deaf. Deaf because the patient is not welcomed as a person and is not even heard. Blind because, by limiting itself to understanding the disease only as an expression of biological variables evidenced by subsidiary tests, it does not recognize the patient as a biographical being. A study carried out to evaluate the doctor-patient relationship in public and private health care services in the city of Londrina revealed the stage of this true relational catastrophe. A total of 647 patients were interviewed, 324 of whom were users of the Unified Health System (SUS) and 323 of private health insurance. The results for patients from the public health system showed: a) patients spent more than 90 minutes in the waiting room before being seen by a doctor: 171 (53.1%); b) users were not called by name during the consultation: 105 (32.6%); c) the consultation lasted less than 10 minutes: 223 (69.9%); d) patients did not undergo a physical examination: 97 (30.2%) (SIQUEIRA, J.E., 2005).

The bond between professional and patient that health augmentations impose must be the result of two complementary movements. The patient who seeks out the professional and the welcome he or she must offer. Both are qualitatively distinct, but Hippocrates found a word to describe them: *"philia"*, which can be translated as friendship, love, solidarity and compassion. For Lain Entralgo, this feeling must necessarily be present in any medical care. To this end, he recalls the words of the great Spanish clinician Gregorio Maranon: *"I have never had, in all its transcendence, an idea of the value of the constitutional element in medicine, as when I read my first clinical histories: those collected with such detail, but with such poor method, in the last years of medical studies and in the first years of professional and hospital life. They described the symptoms, the analyses (chemical and bacteriological) and, sometimes, the lesions, in other words, the illness; but the patient wasn't there. Not one mention of what the person who sustained the illness was like..."* (ENTRALGO, P.L,.1986)

The 20th century brought about the most extraordinary development in biomedical technology, while paradoxically reducing the credibility of doctors. Patients trust technology and distrust professionals. In the same way that they value the information provided by equipment, they underestimate doctors' ability to make accurate diagnostic judgments. Add to this the growing presence of profit-driven private teaching companies, institutions guided exclusively by financial interests, and the end result is the chaos that prevails in health care in our country. A precarious training apparatus, graduates with little regard for social responsibilities and low professional salaries are additional ingredients in the indigestible meal offered by the Brazilian health system.

How can we recover the true Hippocratic *"philia"* in a society that underestimates the exercise of the principle of otherness in medical practice? Lain Entralgo proposes three fundamental principles for bringing doctor and patient closer together in a more harmonious relationship: a) Principle of maximum technical competence: the professional must have a thorough technical training that enables him or her to make sensible use of all the instruments that technoscience offers; b) Principle of the job well done: the doctor must use his intellectual capacity and technical knowledge with the patient's good as his only guide; c) Principle of the authenticity of the good: in situations of moral conflict, the professional must respect the patient's authentic interest according to the values expressed by the patient. (ENTRALGO,P.L., 1983). It is clear that there is a close relationship between the roadmap suggested by Entralgo and the four pillars for educating professionals for the 21st century, as proposed by UNESCO: learning to know, learning to do, learning to be and learning to live together (CIRET-UNESCO, 1997).

There is a long way to go to reach this level, but let's see: in 1996, the Federal Council of Medicine (C.F.M.), the National Federation of Doctors, the Brazilian Medical Association and the Oswaldo Cruz Foundation published an interesting document entitled: "Profile of doctors in Brazil". Volume IV on the data collected in the state of Paraná shows the following results: a) 68.4% of doctors had three jobs, while 31.6% worked four or more jobs; b) 88.1% depended for their personal and/or family subsistence on meager income from agreements with health companies, group medicine or medical cooperatives; c) 82.8% stated that they suffered severe physical and mental exhaustion in the exercise of their profession; d) 65.5% were in favor of strikes in the category, with 5.3% believing that even emergency care should be suspended in this circumstance. These are the final words of the document: *'"In this unfavorable scenario for doctors, the future of the profession is seen by the majority with a strong negative feeling, reflecting the discontent and lack of professional prospects that are now presented to Brazilian doctors."'* (PERFIL DOS MEDICOS NO BRASIL, 1996). As a result of these worrying references, the C.F.M. held the "International Seminar on the Medical Profession" the following year. On the occasion of this event, the President of the Brazilian Medical Association said: "(...) *Quality of care was also another important issue highlighted. What has been happening to doctors all over Brazil for the last two or three years? To the extent that he was able to attend ten appointments for what was theoretically still a good price at the time, and which is now completely devalued, the doctor has chosen a much more comfortable alternative for himself: he doesn't react, he doesn't say that he won't attend, so he has preferred to double the number of appointments with health insurance companies in order to have an adequate financial result. As a result, quality drops. There's no way that a doctor who normally sees ten patients can see twenty patients in one hour. This has a direct impact on the quality [of the service provided]"* (SEMINARIO INTERNACIONAL-PROFISSAO

MEDICA,1997). In 1998, the C.F.M. published "Os medicos e a Saude no Brasil" ("Doctors and Health in Brazil"), which reads: *"Whether it's just a result or a generating factor of the crisis, it doesn't matter, the fact is that the process of training doctors in contemporary society is beset by immense challenges. The technological foundations of practice, the true pillar of medical training today, face the dilemma of producing little benefit for the majority of society, which is excluded from access to them or receives them only marginally. The individualistic appeal, based on the doctor-patient relationship inspired by the Hippocratic oath and generating an artisanal model of service provision that was undoubtedly effective in times gone by, has become a true anachronism. Contemporary medicine is strongly intermediated in institutional, bureaucratic and economic terms and medical schools don't seem to be aware of this fact, carrying out their teaching and care activities as if times were still different."* (OS MEDICOS E A SAUDE NO BRASIL, 1998) These data extracted from surveys carried out by the C.F.M. over three consecutive years speak for themselves. Additional studies carried out in the current century show similar if not more disturbing results. The search for atypical solutions such as the Mais Medicos (More Doctors) Program, which proposed training more professionals to fill the low demand from municipalities lacking doctors, has proven to be fallacious. A recent study carried out by researchers from the University of Sao Paulo (USP), sponsored by the CFM, showed that there had been no significant change in the distribution of doctors across the different regions of the country. (SCHEFFER, M. 2018)

The justification is quite simple and can be summed up in the simple fact that minimum conditions are required to be implemented in municipalities lacking professionals, so that practicing medicine becomes possible. How will it be possible to practice medicine if the doctor does not have the minimum adequate hospital infrastructure or a clinical analysis laboratory that can carry out basic tests to support diagnostic and therapeutic procedures? This was the question that the federal government either didn't ask or didn't want to address before the official program was launched, preferring to adopt a simplistic solution that lacked the foundations to make it a reality. On the other hand, if the process of globalization is inevitable and we are rapidly moving towards the cynical reality of the Minimal State, where the law of the free market and the rule of "save whoever you can" prevail, it is the duty of those responsible to preserve a minimum of morality. If the central government chooses other priorities and decides to shirk fundamental responsibilities such as security, education and health, health professionals cannot fail to identify and clearly denounce who are the perpetrators and victims of this society that globalizes losses and privatizes profits. Few professions enjoy the privilege of being able to share and mitigate human pain and suffering like those involved in health care. Care for the sick can therefore never be animated by an attitude of disrespect or disaffection, because the protagonist of this care is a human being who cannot be treated as an object, because they are an end in themselves and endowed with dignity. This being, whom Boff describes as sacred, the subject of personal history and an essential element in building a more humane society, is capable of living with and dialoguing with the mysteries of the world and asks for the ultimate meaning of life and communes with others, seeing in them the image of the Creator. The essence of the human being's actions, therefore, must always be oriented towards care. (BOFF, L., 1999 a)

Faced with the difficulties pointed out, it is clear that the art of good care has been de-characterized. On the other hand, it is essential to recognize that the individual and the collective are part of the same reality, they are articulated members of the same body. Human beings and society are inseparable entities. Both respond to the same stimuli and, at the same time, suffer the same pains.

If we adopt the rules of the free market as our guide, the incessant search for personal advantage, the logic of the accumulation of goods and contempt for others will prevail. In this way, human beings, fauna, flora and all the riches that surround us lose their intrinsic value and become products to be sold on a huge trading floor Just in passing, we can point to some of the irreversible damage that this model imposes on life on the planet, just by considering the data provided by the UN World Commission on the Environment in 1992. At the time, it was estimated that every year, 6 million hectares of productive land were turned into desert, which meant losing an area equivalent to the territory of Saudi Arabia every 30 years. Every year, more than 11 million hectares of forest were destroyed, which would mean losing the area of India every 30 years (SIQUEIRA, J.E., 1998).

The American scientist Kennet Baoulding described the capitalist model of economy as "cowboy", based on the seemingly unlimited abundance of resources and territories to be enjoyed and invaded according to the Baconian rule of enslaving nature and putting it at the service of man, which constitutes irresponsible and predatory anthropocentrism. (BOFF,L., 1999 b) The logic of the market is oriented towards competition and not cooperation. It is everything, and all of society's problems must be solved in it. This fundamentalism gives centrality to opportunistic and speculative financial capital, which is ruining the economies of emerging countries and making authentically human life impossible. What does this have to do with human health, the subject of this essay? Data from the World Organization for Children in 1998 showed that approximately 250 million children worked in unhealthy conditions, many of them under the age of five. In Latin America, 3 out of 5 children worked; in Africa, 1 out of 3; in Asia, 1 out of 2. The 21st century, as it was awakening, showed us indices of social injustice similar to, if not worse than, those presented so far (BOFF, L., 2001).

Considering the microcosm represented by the human being, we realize that the long reign of Cartesianism in science has banished the qualitative from life and imposed the quantitative. According to Max Weber, the last stage in the improvement of this model is represented by *"specialists without spirit, sensualists without heart, and this nullity imagines that it has reached a level of civilization that has never been reached before".* (RIEFF,P., 1990)

All health professionals recognize that there is no illness that manifests itself outside of a personal temperament, of experiences and experiences already lived and even if it presents itself with a similar physiognomy as a whole, its traces always show in the details, singular colors of the biographical human being. In Foucault's words, *"the sick person is the illness that has acquired singular traits, given with shadow and relief, modulations, nuances, depth, and the task of the health professional, when describing the illness, will be to recognize this living reality"*. (FOUCAULT, M., 1998). Each person falls ill in their own particular way, regardless of how health professionals classify them in this or that nosological category. Each treatment must be unique in the doctor-patient interpersonal construction. Lain Entralgo describes the patient's sense of identity as an integral human being as follows: *"It's my living body that thinks, wants and feels."* (ENTRALGO, P.L., 1996)

For specialists who perceive only their areas of knowledge as real, i.e. the small territory of their knowledge, it is imperative to heed the warning of Marcuse, who described one-dimensional man as one who specialized in a single language and perceived the world only through it.

For him, the expert, *"the world is only what the games of his language register as true. The rest is unreal"*. (MARCUSE, H., 1964). In the real world, people play many games simultaneously: games of love, games of power, games of knowledge, games of pleasure, games of doing, games of playing, games of seduction and even games of getting sick. This is how life is, an endless sequence of games. To perceive it differently is to ignore what is most essential about it (ALVES, R., 2001).

2 BETWEEN VIRTUE ETHICS AND DUTY ETHICS

It is essential to recognize that the 20th century saw substantial changes in the doctor-patient relationship. The first half of the last century was marked by the classic model of virtue ethics, in which the professional, presumably endowed with unquestionable knowledge and vocation, determined the guidelines for the care of the sick. The latter, in turn, passively obeyed the orders imposed on them by the doctors. This characterized an asymmetrical, vertical interpersonal relationship, in which someone with a virtuous education had enough power to impose decisions on others. From the 1960s onwards, the patient began to take on the status of a subject endowed with the capacity to make decisions that best suited him or her, and the role of service provider was reserved for the health professional. Therefore, the ethics of virtue ceased to prevail and the ethics of duty, committed to offering technically correct care, gained importance. In the classical model, the virtuous professional possessed moral perfection by his very nature. This is how a famous Hippocratic aphorism was established: "Where there is love for the sick (*philanthropie*) there is also love for art (*philotekhnie*)". The principle of beneficence therefore prevailed as an expression of the natural practice of virtue ethics. This was the understanding in the Western world for more than twenty centuries. To this end, it is enough to turn to the Oath of Hippocrates, uttered to this day by medical graduates, where the quest for moral perfection can easily be identified with the rules of a private morality for doctors: "I swear by Apollo the physician, by Asclepius, Hygeia and Panacea, as well as by all the gods and goddesses to fulfill (....according to my judgment the oath(...) I will teach this to my children and the children of my masters and to no one else(...) If I fulfill this oath faithfully, I will enjoy my life and my art with a good reputation among men, and forever; but if I depart from it or violate it, the opposite will happen to me."

The new paradigm, on the other hand, subordinated professional decisions to patients' rights, and was therefore guided by the ethics of duty, where the patient's autonomy prevailed in making decisions about the diagnostic and therapeutic approaches to be adopted for their own body, so that it became essential to recognize that patients' rights prevailed over the proposals made by doctors. A contractual relationship was therefore established in which the professionals would offer their knowledge and technical skills and the patient, after receiving the appropriate information, would autonomously make the decisions that would satisfy them most. This transition from the model of virtue ethics to duty ethics has not yet been adequately assimilated by the actors involved in this relationship. The substitution of paternalistic guidance for autonomous decision-making by the patient has had the secondary effect of judicializing the relationship between doctor and patient, transforming health professionals into service providers and therefore subject to legal demands made by patients when they are dissatisfied with the quality of the services provided. By minimizing the decision-making power of professionals, advocates of full patient autonomy argue that only patients are given the right to make decisions about their own bodies. Others, however, consider this new condition in the doctor-patient relationship to be inadequate, as they believe that every human being, when ill, has their decision-making capacity automatically reduced and, above all, they believe that it is impossible for any health professional to transfer to the patient all the information necessary for the best decision-making that each clinical situation requires. There is also a third group that proposes an alternative way of making decisions, inspired by the Habermasian proposal of deliberation, which presupposes respectful dialogue between the parties in the search for consensual solutions that are as reasonable and prudent as possible. The unconditional defenders of the full exercise of the patient's autonomy in making clinical decisions understand that it would be up to the health professional to simply offer technical information, making their skills available to carry out the procedure chosen by the patient. Here, the professional would only play an advisory role, offering all the possible therapeutic alternatives so that the patient could make decisions according to what best suited them. Not unjustifiably, this model has been very well received in countries with an Anglosaxon culture, where extreme respect for the exercise of individual rights is cultivated. In this scenario, the patient goes to the health professional to receive a technical service and everything must be governed by a contract which includes the rights and duties of each of the parties involved in the treatment. In the practice of medicine, this relationship model has generated, on the one hand, lay entities that specialize in identifying possible professional errors and, on the other, so-called defensive medicine that specializes in drawing up contracts that protect professionals from possible lawsuits filed by patients. Obviously, this impasse has had serious consequences for the process of drawing up and obtaining informed consent. It is clear, therefore, that by replacing the Hippocratic-inspired paternalistic model with the unrestricted exercise of patient autonomy, undervaluing the figure of the virtuous professional and adopting a contractual pact as the mediating element between health professional and patient, the perception grew that the so-called Hippocratic *philia* was giving way to the coexistence of moral strangers, a condition presented by Engelhardt as a real reality in post-modern society, where secular morality prevails (ENGELHARDT,T. 1998). In the paternalistic model, the health professional acted as the sole person responsible for the patient, deciding and putting into practice the procedures that he considered most beneficial for the sick person under his care. Although guided by the technical and moral imperatives of serving the patient's best interests, the professional reserved the right to make decisions based on his personal judgment and competence.

Just to emphasize the possible weaknesses of the paternalist and autonomist models, we will present two hypothetical cases of decision-making for hysterectomy in different clinical situations, which are nevertheless quite common in the daily work of health professionals.

Case 1: Mrs. X, 32 years old, married, third pregnancy and referred to the operating room for a caesarean section. During the procedure, after the fetus had been removed, the surgeon noted the presence of a slight uterine myomatosis which, in his opinion, was sufficient to be responsible for the difficult-to-control trans-operative bleeding. The doctor, considering that the couple presumably no longer wished to increase their offspring, decided, after a quick consultation with the patient's husband, to perform a hysterectomy.

Case 2: Mrs. Y, 33 years old, divorced, with a previous diagnosis of mild uterine myomatosis, presents herself to her gynecologist reporting that she suffers a lot from repeated episodes of premenstrual tension and prolonged metrorrhagia, requesting that the professional perform a hysterectomy in order to spare her from the suffering that impairs her quality of life. The professional, although considering that there was no formal indication for the procedure, since there were other therapeutic alternatives, agreed with the patient and proceeded to remove the uterus vaginally without any post-operative complications, which allowed her to be discharged from hospital early. Two years later, for very different reasons, both patients began to express their desire to become pregnant again. Mrs. X, for having lost her third child to accidental drowning in the swimming pool of the building where she lived; Mrs. Y, for her part, having established a new marital relationship with a young widower, began to express her intention of becoming pregnant in order to fulfill the wish of her husband, who understood that the presence of a child would be an essential element to complement the couple's happiness.

In the case of Mrs. X, decision-making followed the paternalistic model, while for Mrs. Y, the doctor agreed to her wishes, even considering that the procedure did not comply with best clinical practice, and in short, the patient's autonomous will prevailed. Just as an exercise in reasoning, let's consider a new route that would precede decision-making and would consist of promoting with patients what we call, in clinical bioethics, a deliberative process. In this model, which we believe to be the most appropriate, doctor and patient, before making a decision, establish a professional dialog, considering all the possible alternatives, taking into account all the risks and benefits involved in each of the therapeutic proposals presented. This is what we might call cooperative decision-making, undertaken by two "moral friends". Although we know that even after a long deliberative process leading up to the hysterectomy decision in both cases, the final options could be the same as those originally adopted, it is imperative to recognize that simply looking at all the possible alternatives could result in other, more reasonable and prudent decisions. For example, if Mrs. X had had the opportunity to properly evaluate and give her opinion on the indication for a hysterectomy, doesn't it seem sensible to imagine that she might have opted to preserve her organ? And what about Mrs. Y, if she had been presented with other proposals for conservative therapy, without coercion and with greater persuasion on the part of the professional, isn't it plausible to consider that she might have accepted them? Regardless of the answers to the above questions, one thing is certain: dialogue conducted with respect and exhausted so that no doubts remain for all the protagonists involved in the cases, seems to be the most appropriate route to reach the most reasonable and prudent decisions possible. This is the model proposed by bioethics for making clinical decisions that take into account the facts arising from scientific research and human values, since evidence-based medicine alone is not enough to determine the instance of **ought,** which occupies the highest level of moral duty. On the other hand, the proper application of the informed consent form in clinical practice is relatively new to us. We can say without worrying that, particularly in Brazil, it is not uncommon for invasive diagnostic procedures or even major surgeries to be carried out without patients being properly informed. It's not uncommon to see, during a routine consultation in the cardiology outpatient department of a university hospital, that the attending doctor, faced with a patient with a median thoracotomy scar, when asked about the type of surgical procedure carried out, receives a brief response from the patient: "I had a valve replaced in my heart". When asked about the model and position of the prosthesis used, the answer is often: "I don't know, the doctor didn't tell me". Obtaining informed consent in a clinic, although a mandatory procedure, should always be done through a proficient and enlightening dialog so that the patient's personal dignity is respected. Modern society demands that health professionals recognize patients' competence to make decisions regarding diagnostic and therapeutic procedures carried out on their own bodies. Unfortunately, there are still frequent attitudes from professionals who consider humble, poorly educated people to be incapable of understanding explanations about medical procedures. They don't manage or even make an effort to truly communicate with the person who, deprived of the most basic rights of citizenship, bows silently before the authoritarian attitude of the professional. Which health professional hasn't heard of a case in which a diabetic patient with obstructive peripheral arterial disease, when asking the vascular surgeon for clarification on the indication for amputation of his leg, received the laconical response: "Please understand that I have studied for over twenty years to know all the details of this surgery, so rest assured and leave it to me to know what is best for you!"

It must be considered, however, that if the paternalistic behavior of the professional who does not recognize the patient's right to make decisions about procedures to be carried out on their own bodies is reprehensible, the "Pilate attitude" of the doctor who simply transfers all decisions to the patient's sphere of responsibility, without having established a prior clarifying dialogue, is equally irresponsible. Health professionals need to recognize that the consent offered by the patient for any procedure will only have moral support if it is preceded by a respectful and enlightening dialogue about all the risks and benefits of the proposed medical indications. Furthermore, the attitude of providing information to the patient, in addition to being carried out in an interactive manner, presupposes that the doctor has adequate knowledge of the patient's biographical history. Modern medicine lives with a significant increase in chronic illnesses and a multitude of diagnostic and therapeutic possibilities, each with its own risks and benefits, which makes the decision-making process very complex. Between the professional's paternalistic attitude and the insufficiently informed patient's decision making lies prudence in the search for the best and most reasonable alternatives identified by both through the deliberative process. Originally inspired as an instrument to allow patients to make free and autonomous choices, there is currently an inadequate practice of considering the consent form as a formal procedure for obtaining an instrument that offers health professionals legal protection against possible lawsuits brought by patients or their families. In addition to providing sufficient and intelligible information, doctors should not allow pressure from family members to determine clinical decisions that meet expectations outside the patient's own interests. On the other hand, the strategy of offering incomplete information to patients in order to make it easier and quicker for them to accept diagnostic or therapeutic decisions that are considered scientifically more preferable from the doctor's point of view is morally unsound. This reprehensible type of manipulation is also practiced by family members who want to have the last word on the treatment to be given to their sick relatives. Known as the "pact of silence", the agreement made between health professionals and family members with the aim of concealing from the patient information that is considered, a priori, to be harmful to the emotional balance of the sick person, is still a common practice. Some professionals call it a pious lie. It should be borne in mind, however, that lying is invariably harmful to the patient, who, deprived of expressing their autonomous decisions, feels disrespected and reduced to the moral condition of being incapable. It is obvious that the professional must be trained to give the patient good news and, to do so, must be guided by protocols established in the medical literature. Many medical schools have already incorporated workshops into their curricula to enable students to give better news. Although some professionals still consider the use of pious lies to be valid, we are a long way from adopting the advice of Gregorio Maranon, who in the 1940s taught his students that: *"The doctor, therefore, must lie, and not only out of charity, but out of the service of health! How often an inaccuracy, deliberately planted in the mind of the sick person, benefits him more than all the drugs in the pharmacopoeia!"* (MARANON, G., 1947)

The patient is not asking for pious lies, but for pious ways of approaching the truth. It is also important to bear in mind that the roadmap in the quest to know the truth differs enormously between people and at different times in their lives. Any illness generates varying degrees of personal insecurity and erects barriers to lucidity, and the health professional cannot fail to recognize them. Both the pious lie and the untimely truth exposed to the patient only show the professional's unpreparedness to establish a respectful intersubjective bond with the patient. Thus, the flow of information in the doctor-patient relationship must be subject to respect for the most vulnerable and materialize in acts of loyalty and authentic partnership and, to this end, there is no other way than through the permanent exercise of the deliberative process to make clinical decisions. It is important to emphasize that it is up to the patient to define the form, pace and limits of the disclosure of information about their illness, and it is up to the professional to be attentive to the doubts and insecurities of the patient and their family. This practice should be carried out with sufficient time for permanent reassessment of all previous decisions and, whenever possible, should be implemented in a consensual manner. There are, however, special situations that do not allow all the stages of this process to be completed and these are those involving urgent care, when it is necessary to quickly install specific care to maintain the vital functions of the sick person. Likewise, the care provided by some specialists in emergency situations, such as anesthesiologists and intensivists, who almost never have enough time to maintain any dialogue with the patient. Finally, another situation that needs to be considered is when the patient, free from any external coercion, spontaneously decides to transfer responsibility for decision-making to the healthcare professional. This type of delegation of power should not be considered a loss of autonomy on the part of the patient. Attention should also be paid to special circumstances in which it is necessary to allow people who are more familiar with the patient's moral values or beliefs, such as those of an ethnic, religious or cultural nature, to take part in the decision-making process, provided that there is the express agreement of the patients themselves. Health professionals should not oppose such contributions. In short, the doctor-patient relationship should be conducted through a unique dialogue that begins with the patient's personal account of their suffering, followed by active listening, careful physical examination, and ending with diagnostic and therapeutic decision-making based not only on the canons of evidence-based medicine, but also taking into account the patient's universe of moral values. It can never be a meeting between a technician and a sick body, but rather a meeting between two people who, although they have different biographical histories, recognize each other as "moral friends" who cultivate mutual respect.

3 A BRIEF REFLECTION ON THE EMERGING PARADIGM

Reflection on the art of care is essential, especially in order to meet the new conditions arising from the transition from the Cartesian model to clinical decision-making based on dialogic ethics. Thinking about the role of each of the characters, health professional and patient, in this new scenario is a necessary task for successful medical care. The word treatment comes from the Greek *"therapeia"* and means service. The art of care, therefore, is expressed in the service provided by the health professional to the patient. The model, which must now be overcome, focuses on care centered on the disease; the emerging paradigm focuses on caring for the whole patient, considering that illness is not restricted to the suffering of an organ, but rather the total suffering of the human being. Undergraduate health courses continue to train specialists in treating people's illnesses, when society is calling for professionals who recognize that any illness that affects a person does so in its biopsychosocial and spiritual totality. Illness must be perceived as a state of imbalance in human health and the true art of caring seeks to re-establish the lost balance.

Rene Descartes is said to have once said that he only needed to be given the displacements and velocities of celestial bodies to be able to construct the Universe. Modern physics, after the revelation of Heisenberg's Uncertainty Principle and Einstein's Theory of Relativity, definitively buried the mechanistic thesis that sought to explain all scientifically observable phenomena in a pragmatic way based on logico-mathematical knowledge. In the field of health, Cartesianism reduced the human being to a set of biological variables compartmentalized into systems and apparatuses: circulatory, respiratory, digestive, neurological, reproductive, etc. Advances in neuroscience have revealed the existence of neurotransmitters, receptors which, through chemical messengers, promote intercommunication between the nervous, immune and hormonal systems, showing that the human being is much more complex than a heap of juxtaposed organs.

In order to better understand this new reality, it is necessary to turn to Edgar Morin's theory of complexity (MORIN,E, 1995). Health professionals must therefore abandon the Cartesian magnifying glass and realize that they will always be faced with the new challenge of recognizing human beings as *"homo systemus"* who see their personal boundaries passing through multiple interactions with other *"homo systemus",* in an immense variety of social environments, events, choices, losses and renunciations and that both health and illness are situations that will remain misunderstood unless all these variables are integrated.

Hans-Georg Gadamer, professor of hermeneutics at the University of Frankfurt, drew attention to the meaning of the word *sprechstunde,* which is made up of *sprechen (to* speak) and *stunde* (time). He understood that the act of caring contained in the encounter between health professional and patient should be guided by the imperative of "time to speak"*: "The disturbance of health is what makes treatment necessary. Part of treatment is dialog. Dialogue promotes the humanization of the relationship between [professional] and patient. Such unequal relationships belong to the most difficult tasks [to be carried out] between human beings (...) The word dialog already implies talking to someone, [who] responds to his interlocutor (...) In any case, in the field of medicine, dialog is not a simple introduction and preparation for treatment, it is already treatment."* (GADAMER, H.G., 2006). Curiously, the emerging paradigm proposed for this millennium, the repository of the most complex advances in technoscience that humanity has ever known in its history, goes by the simple name of **dialog**. After extolling so much hermetic knowledge, we need to prepare ourselves for the time of speaking and listening. In this respect, there is no better way than to return to the model of Socratic *maieutics*, which uses dialog as a search tool to find the truth. To exemplify this route, we return to the very topical dialogue between Socrates and Phaedon on the subject of rhetoric and the medical art:

- *Socrates:* We proceed with rhetoric as with the art of medicine.

- *Fedon:* Why?

- *Socrates:* In both, you have to break down nature, the body on the one hand, the soul on the other, if you wish, not just in a conventional way and on the basis of simple routine, but with art and strength through the use of medicines and nutrition and, in the case of rhetoric, to convey virtue and the conviction you want through good advice and sacred customs.

- *Fedon: Apparently* so, Socrates.

- *Socrates: Do* you believe that you can correctly understand the nature of the soul without understanding the whole of nature?

- *Phaedon:* If Hippocrates the Asclepian is to be believed, without such a procedure we cannot even understand the nature of the body. (PLATO, 1972)

Equally necessary is to learn from the teachings contained in the verses of T.S. Eliot. Separated in time by twenty-four centuries, the philosopher and the poet teach us that in order to exercise the art of care well, it is necessary to return with insight and wisdom to our origins, because only by welcoming the sick human being with empathy will we know how to properly conduct our professional actions:

"We will never stop exploiting

And at the end of all our exploration

It will be getting to the starting point

And the place still recognizes

Just like the first time we saw him.

Through the unknown, remembered door

When the last speck of earth

Left for us to discover

That was the beginning

On the slopes of the longest river

The voice of the hidden waterfall (...)

Hurry now, here, now, always

A condition of absolute simplicity (...)" (T.S.ELIOT,1981)

References

ALVES, R. *Entre a Ciencia e a Sapiencia: o dilema da educagao.* Sao Paulo:

Loyola, 2001

ALVES, R. *The doctor.* Campinas: Papirus, 2003 BOFF, L. *Saber Cuidar.* Sao Paulo: Vozes,1999 a   . *Etica da Vida.* Brasilia : Letraviva,1999 b   . *Principle of Compassion and Care.* Petropolis: Vozes, 2001 CIRET-UNESCO. *Which university for tomorrow? In search of a transdisciplinary evolution of the university.* Locarno : Ciret-Unesco, 1997 DESCARTES, R. *Discurso del Metodo.* Mexico: Parrua, 1984 ENGELHARDT , T. *Fundamentos de Bioetica.* Sao Paulo : Loyola, 1998

ENTRALGO, P.L. *La relacion medico-enfermo.* Madrid : Alianza Editorial,1983   . *Science, Technology and Medicine.* Madrid: Alianza Editorial,1986   . *Being and Conduct of Man.* Madrid: Espasa,1996 FOUCAULT, M. *O Nascimento da Clinica.* Rio de Janeiro: Forense Universitaria,1998

GADAMER, HG. *The hidden nature of health.* Petropolis: Vozes, 2006

GAILLARD, J.R. *O medico do futuro: para uma nova logica medica.* Lisbon: Instituto Piaget, 1995

LOWN, B. *The lost art of healing.* Sao Paulo: JSN Editora,1997

MARANON, G. *Vocation y Etica y otros ensayos.* Madrid : Espasa Calpe,1947

MARCUSE, H. *One dimensional man: studies in the ideology of advanced industrial society.* Boston: Beacon,1964

MORIN,E. *Introduction to Complex Thinking.* Lisbon: Instituto Piaget,1995 THE MEDICS AND HEALTH IN BRAZIL, Federal Council of Medicine .Brasilia,1998 PERFIL DOS MEDICOS NO BRASIL ,vol.IV. Rio de Janeiro, Fiocruz/CFM/MS/PNUD,1996

PLATO *Collection The Thinkers, vol.III.* Sao Paulo : Abril,1972

RIEFF, P. *O triunfo da terapeutica.* Sao Paulo : Editora Brasiliense,1990

ROZENMAN,Y. *Where did good old clinical diagnosis go?* New Engl J Med,336:1435-1438,1997

SCHEFFER,M. *Medical demography in Brazil.* Brasilia : Federal Council of Medicine, 2018

INTERNATIONAL SEMINAR ON THE MEDICAL PROFESSION. Federal

Council of Medicine, Brasilia, 1997

SFEZ,L. *A saúde perfeita: cntica de uma nova utopia* .Sao Paulo : Loyola,1996

SIQUEIRA,J.E. *Etica e Tecnociencia: uma abordagem segundo o Principio de Responsabilidade de Hans Jonas.* Londrina :EDUEL,1998

---------------- . *Bioethics Education in Medical School* The World of Health, year 29,v. 29,n.3,July/September,402-410,2005

T.S.ELIOT *Poetry.* Rio de Janeiro : Nova Fronteira,1981

4 MODERNITY AND THE EMERGENCE OF APPLIED ETHICS

"The challenge for future bioethics is that we possess more technological knowledge than ever before, but we have no sense of how to use it, and the crisis of our age is that we have acquired unexpected power and must use it in the chaos of a post-traditional, post-critical and post-modern world." (ENGELHARDT, T.,1998)

The traditional ethical models that prevailed until the 19th century were characterized by an emphasis on human actions that met the Kantian categorical imperative. The search for the universalization of moral acts carried out by men and women living in communities that were heterogeneous in their customs made it almost impossible to imagine an imperative of human reason that could contemplate the condition of being universal, as proposed by Immanuel Kant (KANT, I., 1985). It took two world wars for us to understand the harsh reality described by Freud as the "death drive", a psychological condition which, according to him, gave human beings obscure desires for self-annihilation, which were externalized through hetero-destruction. In this way, it would be unreasonable to attribute universal moral value to all human acts, since many of them would represent the externalization of the impulse to destroy others, as a substitute for the desire for one's own self-annihilation (FREUD, S., 1981).

Similarly, until the 19th century, nature had real normative power and human freedom was entirely subject to a natural and immutable horizon. From the second half of the 20th century onwards, we began to see that *technical-scientific* advances took on the characteristics of an almost unlimited power to transform human and extra-human natures, entirely subjugating *homo-sapiens* to *homo faber*. On the other hand, the relationship between technology and science became dominant and the product of this union - technoscience - acquired extraordinary powers, producing advances that gained such autonomy that it was considered unnecessary to subject them to any ethical judgment. In a famous lecture on the crisis of European science and transcendental phenomenology, Husserl already identified the existence of a "blind hole" in scientific objectivism, which he then called "*the emptiness of consciousness in itself*". (HUSSERL,E.,1994)

From the moment that, on the one hand, there was a divorce between human subjectivity (reserved for psychology and philosophy) and the objectivity of knowledge (considered to be the exclusive territory of science), the development of refined technologies to unravel the mysteries of nature began to be privileged. This condition was criticized by Morin, who identified it as an "*ignorance of the ecology of action*" (MORIN, E., 1993), since from the moment the process of seeking knowledge begins, the control of the actions that follow it is beyond the control of the researcher and begins to be conducted by agents outside the field of science, who begin to define objectives other than those originally conceived. It would be idle to list examples of this deviation, suffice it to recall that the knowledge generated by the energy released by nuclear fission, among other noble scientific initiatives, enabled the production of the atomic bombs dropped on Hiroshima and Nagazaki.

On the other hand, it is important to recognize that the foundations of modern science have their roots in the 17th century, with Rene Descartes and Francis Bacon, who emphasized the operative power of science. In "De l' Avancement des Sciences", originally published in 1603, shortly before his death, Bacon encouraged men to join forces "*to dominate nature, take by storm and occupy its castles and palaces.*" (BACON, F., 1999). In fact, men of science did everything possible to respond to Bacon's proposal. A new model of collaboration between technology and science was then produced, in such a way that any scientific research would be carried out through an intimate dialog between the search for knowledge and its practical application, between theory and the use of the product it generated.

On the subject, Popper pondered that:

"*The history of science, like that of all human ideas, is a history of irresponsible dreams, stubbornness and mistakes. However, science is one of the rare human activities, perhaps the only one, in which errors are systematically pointed out and, over time, constantly corrected*". (POPPER,K. 1972)

In the 20th century, we came to recognize that in the face of the possibility of damage to human and extra-human nature resulting from technoscientific advances, it was mandatory that, at the same time as producing new knowledge, science should welcome the necessary and prudent contributions of ethical considerations about values that are essential to life. There was no shortage of thinkers like Ralph Lapp, quoted by Alvin Toffler in "The Shock of the Future", who considered it essential to inhibit the uncontrolled advance of technoscience.

Lapp used the following metaphor:

"We are on a train that is constantly gaining speed, running down a track where there are countless steering controls that lead to unknown destinations. No single scientist is in the cockpit and it's possible that there are demons in the control panel. Most of society is in the last seat, looking backwards. (TOFFLER,A. 1973)

More thoughtful was Toffler himself, who considered that turning our backs on technology would be naïve and unwise. What would be important, according to him, would be to define an efficient strategy to avoid what he called the "shock of the future". Gilbert Hottois, a Belgian bioethicist, also considered that *"both the obscurantist rejection and the reckless glorification of technoscience could be harmful to the quality of life of future generations".* It is important to consider that only human beings are capable of changing the course of history through their actions and choices, which need to be subjected to prudent ethical reflection. This responsibility imposes on everyone - especially scientists involved in the production of knowledge - duties that take into account the preservation of human existence in its authentic form. The obligation becomes significantly greater in view of the power of transformation and the awareness we have of all the possible damage caused by ill-considered actions (HOTTOIS, G. 1991).

It is important to consider that only human beings are capable of changing the course of history through their actions. On a road that forks, only the human being has a choice. The routes can be different, as can the final destination, because a path can end at a precipice or at a spring of pure water. It is precisely at these bifurcation points that the question of choice arises, which will only be appropriate if conducted through an interdisciplinary dialogic process involving representatives from all areas of knowledge. This responsibility imposes on all scientists involved in the production of knowledge duties that take into account the preservation of human existence in its most authentic form. The obligation becomes significantly greater as a result of the power of transformation and the awareness we have of all the possible damage caused by ill-considered actions. Maintaining life in its fullness is the condition for human survival, and it is in the context of this solidary destiny that Hans Jonas, author of "The Principle of Responsibility", speaks of the dignity of nature. Preserving nature, according to Jonas, means preserving life in its most genuine expression (JONAS, H. 1995).

In the same vein, we highlight the warning cry of Edgar Morin and Anne Brigitte Kern, described in their book "Terra-patria":

"Here's the bad news: we're lost, irretrievably lost. We're lost, but we have a roof over our heads, a house, a homeland. It is our homeland, the place of our community of destiny, of life and death. The gospel of lost men tells us that we must be brothers, not because we will be saved, but because we are lost". (MORIN, E. KERN,A.B,1995).

Furthermore, the damaging repercussions on human health resulting from the deterioration of the environment are well known. The future may not be realized, but it bears witness in the present, as the characterization of a misfortune, a perspective of the unwanted, which eloquently shows us the need to draw up a new statute of responsibility aimed at maintaining human life and the planet.

Ilya Prigogine, Nobel Prize winner in Chemistry, in his book "The End of Certainties", also lectures on the need for a dialog between science and nature. The author considers that "understanding" cannot mean "controlling", because:

"The master who believed he knew his slaves simply because they obeyed his orders would be blind [...]. No [scientific] speculation, no knowledge has ever affirmed the equivalence between what is made and what is unmade, between a plant that is born,

blossoms and dies, and a plant that resurrects, rejuvenates and returns to its primitive seed, between a man who matures and learns and [the one] who progressively becomes a child, then an embryo, then a cell". (PRIGOGINE, I.,1996).

On the other hand, it is important to recognize that current concerns about ecological imbalance also stem from the almost non-existent system of environmental accounting. The internationally accepted system for recognizing a nation's economic progress, the so-called Gross Domestic Product (GDP), does not take into account the depreciation of "natural capital", such as the loss of fertile soils due to erosion, the indiscriminate use of agrochemicals or deforestation.

Giovane Berlinguer, an Italian bioethicist, in his book "Questions of Life: Ethics, Science and Health", expressed his indignation at the uncontrolled gallop of technoscience: *"The speed with which we move from pure to applied research is now so high that the permanence, even for a short time, of errors or fraud, can cause catastrophes."* (BERLINGUER, G.,1993)

In *"Global Bioethics: building on the Leopold Legacy",* Van Rensellaer Potter, creator of *the* neologism *bioethics, addressed* the issue of responsibility in the search for knowledge. Specifically addressing scientists, he recommended that they *"think of bioethics as a new ethics of science that combines humility, responsibility and competence, that is interdisciplinary and intercultural and that brings out the true sense of humanity."* (POTTER, V.R.,1988).

In the 20th century, we witnessed countless misfortunes, just by considering the human losses accumulated in the two great wars and the degradation of the environment. What paths have we taken that have made us lose our sense of community and let us be dominated by an obstinate and irresponsible individualism? Perhaps because we have chosen the rules of the "isolated self" to represent the superiority of the part over the whole, we have relieved ourselves of all responsibility for understanding and addressing the problems of the human community. Amartya Sen has identified as the most misleading motto of post-modern reflection the fact that we have considered that the supposed virtues of the regulatory mechanisms of the free market have proved to be so obvious that they do not require any ethical reflection to assess their social consequences. The author concludes that capitalism, in trying to show with incomparable richness of detail that the scientifically-based economy should always fluctuate according to the market, did not have the objective of defending democracy, but rather the freedom of movement of big international capital, which recent events have shown has only resulted in a huge increase in social inequalities (SEN, A. 2011).

More recently, the French economist Thomas Piketty published "Capital in the 21st Century", the result of fifteen years of research into the evolution of economic policy in twenty countries over the last two hundred years. In the conclusion of this research, the author states that "*the general link of my research is that the dynamic evolution of a market and private property economy, left to its own devices, contains important forces of convergence, linked above all to the diffusion of knowledge and qualifications, but also forces of vigorous divergence that are potentially threatening to our democratic societies and the values of social justice on which they are founded*" (PIKETTY, T., 2014).

The underestimation of the value of human dignity, coupled with chronic problems such as hunger, poverty, unhealthiness and unemployment, has allowed violence to develop at all levels of society, from the domestic to the communal. This unease has stimulated a great deal of academic production in the search to build models that restore the ideals of solidarity and peace, hard-won achievements of modern democracies. Adela Cortina, like other authors, recovers the Kantian universalist model and Habermas' discursive ethics to propose the construction of a society that enables the existence of minimum levels of justice that are present in global society. He emphasizes that these minimums will not emerge from the liberal political tradition, but through initiatives that promote social inclusion. She warns that an unjust world that underestimates solidarity and fundamental human rights does not meet the minimum conditions for harmonious social coexistence, which would favor the creation of fundamentalist movements that would try to resurrect the old totalitarian regimes and the denial of the democratic conquests so hard won by Western civilization. According to the author, only by overcoming individualism, nepotism and regimes of exception, undoing the borders between countries and strengthening solidarity between peoples would it be possible to achieve social peace. (CORTINA,A 2001) Among us, Schramm and Kottow (SCHRAMM,F.R. KOTTOW,M. 2001), Garrafa and Porto (GARRAFA, V; PORTO,D. 2003) respectively, proposed the "Bioethics of Protection" and the "Bioethics of Intervention", which would assign the state the role of protagonist in initiatives that seek to institute social inclusion policies and socio-political transformations with the aim of emancipating the excluded. Considering these postulates, a question arises: are Western representative democracies capable of implementing these transformations? On the contrary, what we see on a global level is that the levels of extreme poverty, unhealthiness, insecurity, lack of access to food and services are increasing.

education and health, circumstances that only increase the already enormous number of social outcasts. On the other hand, according to Amartya Sen, limiting the concept of poverty to the simple condition of insufficient personal income would be an unacceptable reductionism (SEN.A, 1999), and he believes that the only way to truly promote citizenship is through the emancipation of the socially marginalized.

The lack of references, the crisis of legitimacy of the state and the growth of institutional vacuums that are occupied by organized crime, has only increased the existential disenchantment of people who, taken by fear, lose their sense of identity because they lack adequate social support. Thus, we find ourselves inserted in a globalized society, with significant technological advances, a small number of people with enormous fortunes living together with a huge contingent of miserable people, which has been identified by some authors as the "impoverishing enrichment" of *post-modernity*. The personal identity that should be harmoniously constructed in the richness of cultural diversity has been replaced by the pathetic logic of the "isolated self", as described by Allan Bloom, when referring to American youth:

"The indeterminate future and the lack of a binding past mean that the soul of young people is in a state similar to that of the first men, spiritually naked, unconnected, separate, without inherited or unconditional relationships with anything or anyone. They can be anything they want, but they have no particular reason to be anything in particular. (BLOOM A.,1989)

As a result of this veritable tyranny of the Self, the Other comes to be seen as a foreign element to be disrespected, violated and excluded, which makes the physical destruction of the other increasingly commonplace in large urban centers. An emblematic case of this insane cruelty was the murder of the Pataxo indigenous leader Galdino dos Santos. Summoned to represent his community at a FUNAI meeting, Galdino, without a place to stay, fell asleep on a bench at a bus stop in Brasilia. While he slept, five young middle-class men soaked his body in alcohol and set it on fire. With third-degree burns affecting 90% of his body, the indigenous leader died. In a statement published in the April 21, 1997 edition of Correio Braziliense, one of the young men involved justified the criminal act: *"It was just a joke! We didn't know it was a medium, we thought it was some beggar."* (CORREIO BRAZILIENSE, 1997). The Galdino case forces us to reflect on the authenticity of the much-vaunted feeling of solidarity attributed to the majority of Brazilian citizens, since many of them passively watch such explicit practices of trivializing evil. This testimony shows that the young attackers might not have committed the crime if they had known in advance that the victim was an indigenous leader, because the attack was aimed at a homeless person. On the subject of this crime, Endo refers to a study carried out by UNESCO in Brasilia, which found that in the perception of the middle-class young people interviewed, humiliating transvestites, prostitutes and homosexuals was less serious than graffiti on public buildings, destroying street lamps or traffic signs. In addition, more than 20% of them considered it unjustifiable to impose any punishment as a result of their behavior of mistreating these people. However, individuals who have this kind of attitude should be punished for publicly assuming socially reprehensible attitudes (ENDO, P., 2005).

At a time when economic globalization is tearing down all national borders, the world is living with unbearable levels of poverty, hunger and the most persistent violation of human rights. Just look at the iniquitous treatment meted out to the thousands of Syrian refugees who, fleeing war, seek refuge in the countries of Western Europe. The challenge of recreating an ethic of responsible solidarity in order to "humanize humanity" has never been more urgent. It is against this backdrop of disenchantment that applied ethics has emerged, including bioethics, which is concerned with proposing reflections that seek viable alternative solutions to the moral conflicts that emerge from this situation of social chaos.

5 THE THEME OF RESPONSIBILITY AS SEEN BY CONTEMPORARY THINKERS

In "Politics as a vocation", Max Weber made a distinction between "ethics of conviction" and "ethics of responsibility", considering that, in the case of the former, the ends would justify the means of all human actions (an assumption defended by Marxist thinkers); in the case of the latter, the Kantian tradition of universalizing moral actions would be revived. Weber makes the following comments on the two models:

1. Human life would include different fields of axes where there would be tension between morality, politics and religion, which he recognized as sources of unsolvable conflicts and that the prudent attitude would be to accept them naturally and that no one could be given the right to use a position of superiority to impose their personal convictions on others.

2. All human beings should be responsible for the foreseeable consequences of their actions. In this respect, he puts forward his view that when the consequences of an action carried out out of pure conviction turn out to be unpleasant, the supporter of such an ethical model would not consider the agent who carried it out to be guilty, but rather other random variables such as *"the world, the foolishness of men or the will of God, who created men in this way". On the* other hand, the supporters of the ethic of responsibility would consider that the responsibility for the acts practiced would lie exclusively with the agent who practiced them, and it would be unreasonable to transfer the harmful consequences of their own actions to others.

3. The ethic of responsibility would presuppose that the means should be appropriate to the ends to be achieved and that there could be no altruistic ends that would justify resorting to means that are incompatible with the realization of the authentic objectives of the original goals (WEBER, M.1980).

Likewise, in "Essay on axiological neutrality in the sociological and economic sciences", published in 1917, Max Weber makes a distinction between obtaining the facts produced by science and the possible evaluations of value resulting from them.

At the time, what mobilized the attention of the academic community was the question of "freedom of professorship", a condition that gave professors total freedom to express personal judgments on matters in their field of knowledge. Weber, however, argued that any argument that could justify the superiority of any professor's particular point of view over those defended by other thinkers would be disproportionate in matters of politics and social coexistence. He considered that it would be immoral for teachers to use their hierarchical position to influence or even indoctrinate their students. At the same time, the German intelligentsia was passionately debating the theoretical question of the social sciences, and there was a real dispute between those who defended the adoption in this area of knowledge of the same methodological rigors used in investigations carried out in the field of natural sciences, which were markedly quantitative. On the other hand, other thinkers considered it essential to include subjective values in this area of research and not just the facts obtained from experiments carried out in the field of exact sciences. It is important to consider that the production of knowledge until the first half of the 20th century was heavily influenced by the positivist philosophy proposed by Auguste Comte, who saw sociology as a field of science capable of explaining social phenomena in an entirely rational manner. By dispensing with the incorporation of subjective values, it limited sociological research to the simple task of purely describing social phenomena, which made dialogue between science and philosophy an almost impossible task. For a long time, this was how the production of knowledge proceeded, in the restricted analytical and quantitative territory, a condition that placed qualitative research in the barely respectable field of academic initiatives of questionable scientific value. However, Max Weber did not consider there to be any incompatibility in simultaneously accepting quantitative and qualitative parameters in scientific research.

In "Protestant Ethics and the Spirit of Capitalism", originally published in 1905, Weber studied the most diverse human behaviors that brought Protestant ethics and the rationalism present in the capitalism of the post-industrial era closer together.

At the time, it was common to compare the perceptions of values that differentiated the behavior of Catholics and Protestants, with the former underestimating the lucrative activities of the business model, while Protestants adopted opposite positions, which were defined by Weber as the *"search for the joy of living"*. According to the author, this perception was not part of the original message of Lutheranism, but was incorporated later as a result of a historical process called ascetic vocation, a condition which advocated that the true meaning of human life was dependent on a divine predestination, in which the accumulation of material wealth would only identify the people chosen by God to demonstrate his manifestation among men. Weber's thesis found support in the writings of Richard Baxter, an important figure in Methodism, who preached that idleness was the greatest expression of sin against God and that in order to be sure of his state of grace, every man should work tirelessly to demonstrate his worthiness in the face of divine grace.

Baxter advised that true believers should work, save and get rich, because only in this way could they both demonstrate their personal merit and ensure their eternal salvation by resisting idleness and pleasure. In this way, Max Weber sought to establish a direct link between puritanism and capitalism (WEBER, M., 2008). Some sociologists have considered that Weber's hypothesis was presumably confirmed by the fact that the main founders of the English chemical industry were Calvinists.

Well, what does this Weberian thesis have to do with the aim of this essay? To answer this question, we need to compare the political ideas that guide the public actions of two countries, one of which is mostly Protestant and the other with the largest number of devout Catholics on the planet. We are talking about the USA and Brazil. To this end, we will consider the thinking of two contemporary philosophers, Robert Nozick and Franklin Leopoldo e Silva. In 1974, Nozick published "Anarchy, State and Utopia", in which he questioned the validity of the concept of distributive justice, arguing that individual rights are so inalienable and comprehensive that no democratic government would be authorized to allocate public funds from income taxes to social programs aimed at benefiting poor people, without them making their own contributions to the state coffers. According to the author, attitudes of this nature would only favor the maintenance of the state of inertia of this population of indigent people who would no longer exercise their social responsibilities by passively waiting for the benefits provided by a paternalistic government. For him, only a "minimal state", limited to enforcing contracts and providing security for people against arbitrariness, theft and fraud, would be justified in a liberal society. Thus, for Nozick, any government that used the power granted to it by the taxpayers' vote should be prevented from implementing welfare programs for the needy. Thus, one of the premises that a democratic country should adopt as a petrea clause would be not to oblige any citizen to do anything that is not of their own free will, including financial contributions to benefit needy people who may exist in the community (NOZICK, R.1974). This political idea is still prevalent in American society. Evidence of this is the intransigent opposition of the Republican Party to the initiatives of the Barack Obama administration in an attempt to implement proposals that guarantee medical care for a significant proportion of people living in the USA who do not have a health insurance plan: a condition that is extremely costly in that country's health insurance market. We are talking about a population of around 40 million people, a huge contingent of individuals who do not have health insurance and are therefore prevented from enjoying the benefits of access to high-tech procedures in the country that has the best health care services in the world. Franklin Leopoldo e Silva, for his part, analyzes the crisis of reason and applied ethics in "Da etica filosofica a etica em saude" (From philosophical ethics to ethics in health), with special emphasis on bioethics and its expression in human health, arguing that the new discipline would be a useful instrument for answering questions about the relationship between science and human values. According to him, this crisis was caused by historical circumstances linked to the overestimation of profit to the detriment of the feeling of solidarity with the most vulnerable. It is important to remember that, according to the precepts of Kantian ethics, human dignity could not be assigned a price. For the author, there is no justification for a person to suffer inequitable or degrading conditions in their personal life, especially in the area of health. In concluding his exposition, Franklin addresses all those who have responsibility in the health area: *"It is necessary to know the reality [of social deprivation] and the situations in which ethical judgment is to be exercised, but to make this judgment a mere justification of what exists is to renounce ethics"* (LEOPOLDO E SILVA, F. 1998). In this way, it is possible to see that the distance that separates the Brazilian philosopher's thinking from that defended by the American Nozick, is inversely proportional to that which brings him closer to the *one-to-another* ethics of the French philosopher Emmanuel Levinas, whose thinking we will briefly present later in this essay. (LEVINAS,E. 1993)

Hans Jonas, a German philosopher who died in 1993, introduced the figure of the "heunstics of fear" to justify the adoption of a prudential attitude in the face of the moral uncertainties generated by techno-scientific interventions. The author identified the production and subsequent dropping of the atomic bombs on Hiroshima and Nagasaki as a milestone in the inappropriate use of technology. Jonas, in an interview published in Esprit magazine in May 1991: *"It set thinking in motion towards a new kind of questioning, ripened by the danger that our power represents for ourselves, the power of man over nature."* (GREISCH,J. 1991).

Rather than being aware of an abrupt apocalypse, Jonas recognized the possibility of a gradual apocalypse resulting from the reckless use of technological advances. The author pondered that until the 20th century, the scope of ethical prescriptions was restricted to interpersonal human relations. It was an anthropocentric ethic focused on a specific historical moment. Techno-scientific intervention, following the mastery of nuclear physics, has drastically changed this simple reality, subjecting nature to human designs, in other words, it can be radically altered, a condition which now requires the creation of a new pact of responsibility between man and nature. Jonas concludes by saying that this new ethical proposition should consider the harmonious coexistence between man and extra-human nature.

The author stated that all previous traditional ethics obeyed three premises characterized by the following presuppositions:

1. Human and extra-human conditions, regardless of human intervention, have always remained unchanged.

2. Based on the above assumption, one could clearly and without any difficulty determine the good of human and extra-human nature.

3. Responsibility for human actions and their consequences would be perfectly delimited in time.

Nature would not be protected by human actions, because it would be able to take care of itself. Ethics had to do with the here and now. In place of the old ethical imperatives, including the Kantian norm: *"Act in such a way that the principle of your action can become a universal law",* Jonas proposes a new imperative: "Act in *such a way that the effects of your action are compatible with the permanence of authentic human life"* or, to put it negatively, *"Do not endanger the indefinite continuity of humanity on Earth."* (JONAS, H. 1995). The tremendous vulnerability of nature subjected to techno-scientific intervention became an unusual situation, since nothing less than the entire biosphere became susceptible to being altered, making it essential to consider that not only the human good should be sought, but also that of all extra-human nature. Furthermore, new interventions transforming the very nature of the human being revealed the proportions of the challenge for ethical reflection. Jonas listed a series of questions in different areas of human health, for example, with regard to the use of disproportionate medical procedures aimed at artificially prolonging human life, known as dysthanasia, he asks: To what extent is this justified? Regarding the control of human conduct, would it be ethical to induce feelings of happiness or pleasure in people's lives using chemical stimuli? With regard to genetic manipulation, where man has taken the evolution of his own species into his own hands, the philosopher asks: is man prepared for the role of Creator? Who would be the sculptors of the new image of the human being, according to what criteria and based on what models? Does man have the right to alter his own genetic heritage?

The philosopher warned: *"Faced with the almost eschatological potential of our technology, ignorance of the ultimate consequences is in itself sufficient reason for responsible moderation [...]. There is another aspect worth mentioning: the unborn lack power [...]. What forces should represent the future in the present?"* (JON AS, H. 1995). Faced with such an extraordinary power of transformation, Jonas understood that we are devoid of moderating rules to order our actions. This enormous maladjustment could only be corrected, in the author's view, by formulating a "new ethic". With regard to the environment, Jonas considered that *"the responsibility instituted by nature, that is to say, that which existed by [its own] nature, would be independent of our prior agreement. [It would be an irrevocable, uncancellable and global responsibility."* (JONAS,H. 1995). He understood that in the era of a civilization dominated by technology, man's first duty would be to his own future. And respect for the environment as a "sine qua non" condition for the maintenance of human life would already be clearly contained therein. We should therefore bear in mind that the exuberant and sophisticated life of the planet, which has been achieved through a long period of creative work and is now dependent on human intervention, demands a new commitment from all of humanity to protect and preserve a healthy environment.

With a similar perception, Morin and Kern spoke about the relationship between humanity and planetary life:

"the tiny humans on the tiny film of life that covers a tiny planet lost in a huge universe. But at the same time, this planet is a world, life is a pulsating universe of billions and billions of individuals [...] Our terrestrial genealogical tree and our identity card can finally be known today, at the end of the fifth century of the planetary era. And it is precisely now, at the moment when societies spread across the globe are communicating, at the moment when the destiny of humanity is being collectively played out, that they acquire meaning for us to recognize our earthly homeland." (MORIN, E. KERN, A.B., 1995)

The fact is that the conventional economic accounting used by experts values technical progress and underestimates environmental degradation, which ends up allowing the implementation of policies that are predatory to ecological balance. The system for evaluating the different manifestations of life on the planet is quite precarious and we have no idea of the number of species of plants and animals that become extinct every year as a result of untimely human actions. The environmentally destructive interventions introduced in recent decades have resulted in a reduction in agricultural land and uncontrollable environmental pollution. As a result of these problems, spending on projects to decontaminate water sources and on the treatment of illnesses such as skin cancer, various forms of allergy, pulmonary emphysema, bronchial asthma and other respiratory diseases is increasing (SIQUEIRA, J.E., 1998). The inability to adapt non-aggressive technology to the sensitive life of the planet is changing a reality that has lasted for millions of years and generating destruction of the ozone layer, as well as unsatisfactory human development, which is accompanied by poverty and social inequality. There is therefore a link between environmental degradation and social injustice. The absolute figures show that there are currently more people in the world suffering from hunger than ever before in human history. The gap between rich and poor nations is widening and there are no satisfactory indicators to correct this sad reality. (WORLD COMMISSION ON THE ENVIRONMENT AND DEVELOPMENT, 1992).The longevity indices for the Japanese are close to 80 years, while those for the inhabitants of sub-Saharan Africa do not reach 50 years of life.

The fact is that the changes now being introduced into the environment are cumulative and the agents responsible for these transformations will no longer be around for centuries to come to answer for their actions. Future generations have not delegated powers to the current ones for these abstruse decisions, and will only reap the bitter fruits of them. The majority of today's leaders will not witness the most serious effects of acid rain, the global increase in the planet's temperature, the reduction of the ozone layer, uncontrollable desertification and the irreparable loss of its biodiversity. In a public statement, while still President of the United States, Barack Obama warned that the current human generation is the first to feel the harmful effects of environmental degradation and may be the last to adopt measures to save the planet from a disaster of unimaginable proportions. Donald Trump, the current US president, unfortunately thinks otherwise. For him, global warming is a great invention of idle scientists.

We are used to living with problems of limited moral complexity that do little to enable us to understand the disturbing dimensions of the ethical questions that are now being asked. Technoscience only sees black and white, where ethics perceives gray and its different shades. Faced with these questions, Jonas said: "As a result of the inevitably utopian scale of modern technology, the salutary distance between everyday issues and extreme issues, between occasions that call for ordinary prudence and occasions that call for profound wisdom, is shrinking by leaps and bounds [...]. If the new nature of our actions requires a new ethic of long-term responsibility, co-extensive with the range of our power, it also requires, in the name of that same responsibility, a new kind of humility. A humility that is not the same as before, in other words, that is no longer humility in the face of smallness, but rather in the face of the excessive magnitude of our power, which translates into the excess of our power to act [...]. In view of the eschatological potential of our technological processes, ignorance of the ultimate implications itself becomes a reason for responsible restraint [in our actions]." (JONAS, H. 1995).

6 RESPONSIBILITY FOR THE ACT OF CARING INTRINSIC TO THE PRACTICE OF MEDICINE :

"There comes a time when you have to give up used clothes that already have the shape of your body

and forget our paths that always lead us to the same places.

It's time to cross over and if we don't dare to do it, we will have remained on the margins of ourselves forever. " (PESSOA, F.,2008.)

Emmanuel Levinas, born in Lithuania, emigrated to France, where he studied philosophy, delving into the field of phenomenology with Husserl and Heidegger. He taught at the Universities of Poitiers, Paris-Nanterre and finally at Sorbone. Uncomfortable with the rationalism of modernity, which privileged the exaltation of the *"I"*, *he* dedicated himself to reflecting on the importance of the *Other,* inspiring the philosophical current known as the "ethics of alterity". Levinas rejects the understanding of the subject as a monad and his entire philosophical project should be understood as the quest to think from an opening that breaks the monadic structure that modernity has attributed to the human being (LEVINAS, E., 1993). According to the author, only the figure of the *one-for-the-other* would offer a satisfactory answer to the disturbing question posed in the book of Genesis, when God asks Cain about the whereabouts of his brother Abel and receives the evasive answer: "Am I my brother's keeper?" (THE JERUSALEM BIBLE, 2009). Levinas believes that each human being is assigned the task of being responsible for the *Other,* especially those who are socially more vulnerable. According to him, the human community would only survive if it devoted its attention to exercising fraternity and solidarity towards the suffering *Other.* The philosopher is forceful in stating that there is only one possible movement in the life of any person, and that is to go outside oneself in order to reach out to the *Other.* This movement requires radical generosity, because it means moving unconditionally towards the encounter with the *Other,* without any expectation of reward for the merit of this action. Levinas states that this action should be seen as "a work without remuneration", and that the driving force behind it should be otherness, the most complete representation of ethics itself. He pondered that this movement should seek to overcome its own epoch, its own ego, because surrendering to the epiphany of the face of the *Other* would characterize an office that was not only free, but that would require those who exercised it to "give something away". He asked: *"Where does this shock come from when I pass indifferently under the gaze of the Other?"*. Levinas replied: *"The relationship with the Other questions me, empties me of myself and never ceases to present me with ever new possibilities of attending to Him. No, I knew I was so rich, but I no longer have the right to keep anything [for myself]"*. According to him, the *Other* would manifest himself in the face, as an interpellating being, the face would speak and articulate the primordial discourse summoning us to the liturgy of unconditional surrender. The face of the *Other* would impose itself on us without us being able to remain impassive to its appeal, without us being able to claim irresponsibility for the suffering that emerges from it. Faced with the demands of the *Other,* the *Self* would lose the right to remain oblivious. The philosopher adds,

"The epiphany of the absolutely Other is represented by his face which challenges me and [imposes] an order on me [to attend to] his nakedness, his indigence. Its presence [in itself] consists of undoing the very egoism of the "I". Thus, in the relationship with the face [of the Other] the retention of the ethical orientation is delineated". (LEVINAS, E., 1993)

Hopefully, health professionals will be receptive to the voice of Levinas and can be guided by it in caring for their patients. Bioethical reflection is also part of this roadmap in the search for excellence in the practice of medicine. In the article "Bioethics: Science of Survival", Potter defines bioethics as an instrument to be used in order to overcome the demanding reflexive limits provided by academic disciplines, offering thinkers new possibilities for interdisciplinary constructions that facilitate the birth of a "science for the survival of the human species". (POTTER, V.R.1970).

In the health sciences, the need to humanize the relationship between doctor and patient has long been proposed. In the second half of the 20th century, the Spanish clinician Pedro Lain Entralgo taught that "*the professional who wishes to practice medicine as an art should be trained in the humanities*." (ENTRALGO, P.L.1983)

In the context of clinical decision-making, there has always been an asymmetry between professional knowledge and the passivity of the patient in unrestricted acceptance of the advice suggested by those with technical knowledge. This condition of relational asymmetry became known as medical paternalism and remained untouched until the patients themselves, dissatisfied with the little attention they were given, began to assume the condition of autonomous agents, capable of making decisions about their own bodies. During clinical discussions, there was only room for obedience to deontological norms, a territory of moral precepts defined by the medical corporation itself in its professional codes. With a well-defined framework of rules - which could not be questioned - teachers presented students with rules of medical conduct to be followed without it being necessary to take into account the moral values or beliefs of the patients. This model of attitude, captive to norms, characterized a situation of moral immobility that transformed professionals and patients into hostages of deontological instruments that forced them to remain stationary in the uncomfortable condition of moral inferiority. In these circumstances, it was not uncommon for many students to consider it a pointless exercise to discuss clinical cases involving moral conflicts, arguing that there would be no plausible justification for doing so in view of the obligation to obey the rules contained in the deontological codes in force.The Cartesian-Flexnerian model of teaching and medical paternalism therefore appeared to be inadequate tools for training students for the difficult task of helping patients and their families to make decisions in the face of increasingly complex moral conflicts.

If the basic moral character of medical students is to be considered partially structured even before they enter medical school, it is imperative to recognize that a significant part of their ethical formation can be acquired and enriched during the undergraduate period. The Cartesian model divided the complex unity of the human being into smaller and smaller pieces of knowledge and gave the numerous autonomous disciplines the task of constructing medical knowledge. As a result, the period of academic instruction became an obsessive exercise in "accumulating and piling up" information without the slightest concern for selecting and organizing it. In Morin's view, the university would be training professionals with a *full head,* when, on the contrary, it should be preparing them to have a *well-made head,* because more important than the indiscriminate accumulation of scientific information, it would be fundamental to organize it through interactions with other knowledge, in such a way that knowledge could acquire meaning (MORIN, E., 2001).

Concerned about the extraordinary advance of scientific knowledge and the significant growth in the number of academic disciplines, UNESCO set up the International Commission on Education for the 21st Century which, together with the International Commission for Transdisciplinary Research and Studies, drew up the CIRET-UNESCO Project. In the concluding document issued by the organizations, it can be read that "disciplinary research concerns at most a single level of reality [...] fragments of a single level of reality [...] transdisciplinarity is interested in the dynamics generated by the action of several levels of reality simultaneously [...] feeding on disciplinary research [...]. In this sense, disciplinary and transdisciplinary research would not be antagonistic, but complementary." The final report proposes a new type of university education built on the following foundations: learning to know, learning to do, learning to live together, learning to be (PROJETO CIRET-UNESCO, 1997).

In the early 1970s, Andre Hellegers, the first director of the Kennedy Institute of Bioethics, stated that the problems facing doctors in the years to come would be increasingly ethical and less technical. The extraordinary growth of technological medicine was unaccompanied by essential ethical reflection, which led Potter to suggest criteria on when **not to** use all available medical technology in making clinical decisions in the care of terminally ill patients (POTTER, V.R., 1971).

It is imperative to recognize that the unthinking use of technological advances in medicine does not always provide satisfactory results or make them free of moral conflicts. A paradigmatic example of this situation occurred in the USA in 1989, involving an infertile couple who, in their quest to achieve their dream of having a child, sought assistance from an assisted human fertilization clinic. The woman, Luanne, had extensive endometriosis and could not have an embryo in her uterus without the pregnancy becoming high-risk and resulting in an early miscarriage. John, her husband, had oligospermia and sperm with anatomical and functional imperfections. These initial difficulties were overcome by purchasing gametes from anonymous donors, a procedure exempt from unlawful US legislation. Unable to receive the embryo from the "in vitro" fertilization in their own uterus, the couple agreed to hire a healthy woman to be a surrogate mother, under a contract that stipulated the value of US$10,000.00 if the pregnancy was successful, a condition that also had legal support in that country. During the eighth month of pregnancy, the Buzzanca couple divorced and the original agreement was contested by Jonh, who, using the argument that he had no biological link with the product of the pregnancy, felt he was not obliged to take on the paternity of the child. The fetus had already been given the name Jaycee, chosen after the sex of the child had been identified, this information having been provided by an abdominal ultrasound carried out on the surrogate mother in the first weeks of her pregnancy. The disagreement between John and Luanne turned into a legal dispute and the case was referred to the California Supreme Court. After the girl's birth and pending a final court decision, Judge Robert Monarch chose to identify her as "a child without defined parents". Jaycee remained under the guardianship of the State of California for four years, until the final decision of the State Supreme Court won the case for Luanne and, only then, was her parental identity recognized. She came to be recognized as Luanne's daughter, knowing, however, that before the courts of justice she had been denied paternity by John, her sentimental father. Furthermore, Jaycee knew that as well as being the subject of a legal dispute, she would have future difficulties in knowing her biological parents, protected as they were by the secrecy of anonymity, a condition guaranteed by a contract signed between the gamete donors and the fertilization clinic used by the couple for the procedure. (REVISTA VEJA;1998). In the case described, it can be seen that when the medical procedure was carried out, all attention was focused on the interests of the Buzzanca couple, disregarding those relating to the future of Jaycee, the product of the pregnancy ordered by her sentimental parents. The Italian Bioethics Commission, when dealing with the issue of assisted human fertilization, rightly issued the following opinion on 17 June 1994: *"The good of the unborn child must be considered the central criterion for evaluating the various opinions on procreation [...]. Furthermore, it is a fundamental principle that the birth of a human being is the result of a responsibility explicitly assumed with worldwide relevance by those who resort to assisted reproduction. "* (BERLINGUER, G., 2004).

If, on the other hand, we consider the daily routine of medical care, we will conclude that the symptoms that bring the patient to a consultation invariably carry a significant amount of uncertainty, express messages that need to be properly deciphered, which obliges the professional who hears them to be careful in the recommendations they make to the patient. In addition, neuroscientific evidence indicates that when faced with any illness, human beings assume a new existential condition that results from a complex sum of sensations related to the reception, interpretation and representation of their personal vulnerabilities. This condition has been very well analyzed by Susan Sontag in her book "Illness as Metaphor", in which the author describes the impact of illness on people's lives: "Illness *is the dark side of life, a costly citizenship. Although we all like to use only the good passport, sooner or later, each of us is obliged, at least for a while, to identify ourselves as citizens of that other group" (SONTAG,* S., 1984).

This gives us a better understanding of the importance of training professionals who are well prepared in the four areas of mastery proposed by Unesco. In other words, it is not enough for them to have theoretical knowledge or technical skills, but that they know how to *live* and *be in* the community that surrounds them. It is therefore necessary to recognize the relevance of Fernando Pessoa's teachings, when he states in his verses that there is a moment when it becomes necessary to abandon the clothes that have already taken the shape of our bodies and hold us captive to an obsolete model of medical teaching and that we must forget the paths that lead us to the same places as always and that we need to dare to seek the other shore of ourselves in order to reach the other, As Levinas teaches us, this is the only way to fulfill the Hippocratic precept that "where love of man is present, love of art will also be present" (CAIRUS, F.H.;RIBEIRO JUNIOR,W.2005)

Some people's belief that science has the answers to everything stems from a distorted view of reality. We need to be aware of the fact that technoscientific advances bring risks as well as benefits. In medicine in particular, risks and benefits are the common denominator when it comes to applying the extraordinary advances in weaponized medicine and therapeutics. It is essential to always maintain a critical spirit, recognizing that it is unwise to hold back the advances of biomedicine and, at the same time, recognizing that it is unreasonable to cultivate an uncritical optimism that ignores the risks they contain.

It is possible to consider scientific knowledge as important cumulative facts, however, the same cannot be said about the construction of ethical values. Ethics should not be considered as a simple seasoning with the aim of giving a better flavor to the delicacies displayed on the menu of technoscience, but, on the contrary, it is an indispensable ingredient to make the food produced by it healthier for human consumption. We are often overwhelmed by the allure of techno-science and have the illusion that the accumulation of knowledge is enough to make us happy and master the secrets of life. We need to heed Nietzche's forceful sentence about scientism:

"You are cold beings, who feel that you're being encouraged against passion and chimera. You would like your science to become an adornment and an object of

pride! You affix to yourself the label of realist and imply that the world is truly made as it seems to you." (NIETZCHE, F., 2001).

Stopping science from advancing is completely foolish, innocuous and strictly against the essence of human nature, whose aspiration will always be to build new realities. However, it is unreasonable to consider, as some positivists propose, that the man of the techno-scientific age should apply the knowledge he has acquired without any kind of social control. On the contrary, Giovanni Berlinguer ponders that: *"The speed with which we move from pure to applied research is now so high that the permanence, even for a short time, of errors or fraud can cause catastrophes"* (BERLINGUER, G., 2004)..) If, on the one hand, we have the followers of the Baconian precept - which states that the mere fact of mastering knowledge is enough to authorize us to use it in the way that best suits us - on the other hand, we can hear more prudent voices such as Potter, who defined bioethics in his book "Bioethics:bridge to the future": *"My knowledge is limited, but I will combine it with the knowledge and opinions of other intelligent men, inspired by the sense of ethics, and coming from various disciplines, to order my convictions and auguries"* (POTTER, V.R.,1971). Fortunately, between "laissez-faire" and the "satanization" of technoscience, we are offered the sensible path of prudence. The impressive growth of medical technology has been inappropriately assimilated into professional practice, as it has turned from complementary into essential. The ability to collect elucidating anamneses has been greatly diminished, and the detailed physical examination has become a tiresome and even unnecessary exercise in the face of the inexhaustible power of the information provided by the equipment. Technological medicine has changed the way the diagnosis is made and, consequently, the therapeutic act. Medicine, originally a rich art of intersubjective relationships, has been reduced to a poor craft of reading variables provided by equipment. We listen without hearing, because we have been trained to underestimate the expressions of patients' subjectivity. Visits to wards in many university hospitals became a monotonous sequence of reading an endless list of ancillary tests (KANH, 1988). Similarly, with the development of multicenter clinical trials involving large numbers of patients who are followed up for long periods of time, the illusion has been created that the results obtained should become the only guide for the therapeutic conduct of health professionals. However, in doing so, doctors fail to consider that these large "trials" do not necessarily relate to the actual cases they deal with in their daily routines. It is necessary to consider that these studies reveal statistical data referring to a sample of research subjects from all over the world and that simply transposing the information from these studies to particular contexts is a serious mistake that professionals should not make (BOBBIO, M., 2014).

With regard to the inadequate use of diagnostic research methods, Bernard Lown, one of the most renowned cardiologists of the 20th century, described that, of one million *coronary* angiographies carried out in 1993 in the USA, two hundred thousand were normal, and concluded that *"if the guidelines of his master, Prof. Samuel Levine, had been followed, few patients with normal coronary arteries would have been subjected to such an invasive and expensive study"* (LOWN, B., 1996).

Another area where technology has made important contributions to saving lives, but has also led to the adoption of inappropriate procedures, has been the Intensive Care Unit (ICU). It is unnecessary to emphasize the benefits provided by the new diagnostic and therapeutic methodologies, since countless lives have been saved in critical situations, such as the recovery of patients with acute myocardial infarction and/or diseases with severe hemodynamic disorders, whose recovery can only be achieved with the use of ingenious therapeutic procedures. It so happens that our I.T.U.'s have also started to receive patients with incurable chronic diseases, presenting the most diverse clinical conditions, who have been given the same care as the acutely ill. While the latter often achieved a satisfactory recovery, the chronically ill were offered little more than precarious survival, often limited to a vegetative state of life. To what extent should it be considered pertinent to introduce technological artificial life support procedures for patients with incurable diseases?

Traditional medical courses are prodigious at teaching students a lot about cutting-edge technology and little about the transcendent meaning of human life. (SIQUEIRA, J.E.,2005) We have lost the ability to understand the dimension of the teaching contained in the aphorism: "medicine is meant to cure sometimes, relieve very often and comfort always". Doctors are educated to interpret life as a strictly biological phenomenon and use all biomedical technology to pursue this vain utopia. The obsession with maintaining biological life at any cost has led us to therapeutic obstinacy. We therefore have a serious ethical dilemma that is exposed to intensive care doctors on a daily basis when they are forced to decide under what clinical circumstances it is necessary **not to** use all the technology available in the ICU?

7 SOME CONSIDERATIONS ON THE THEME OF DEATH-TABOO

Curiously, "The Economist" magazine, one of the most respected international publications on economics, has, in recent years, been the news outlet that has given the most publicity to articles on end-of-life care. In 2010, it published a report commissioned by the Lien Foundation entitled "Quality of death: the ranking of end-of-life care in the world" (THE ECONOMIST & LIEN FOUNDATION, 2010). The 2015 Report also updated the quality of death index, taking into account the number of palliative care units in the world (THE ECONOMIST & LIEN FOUNDATION, 2015). More recently, in April 2017, in partnership with The Henry J. Kaiser Family Foundation, the journal published a new report entitled: "Visions and experiences with medical end-of-life care in Japan, Italy, the United States and Brazil" (THE ECONOMIST & THE HENRY J. KAISER FAMILY FOUNDATION, 2017). Given the importance of the 2017 report, we will highlight some data that we believe to be essential. The study should merit the attention of all professionals working in the field of chronic and end-of-life care, as it brings to light valuable information about this complex area of medical care. Initially, we will consider patients' opinions on how they would like to be cared for at the end of their own lives. We chose five questions that we felt were the most emblematic: 1. "When it comes to assistance and care, what do you consider most important at the end of your own life?" The answers were: a) prolonging life as long as possible: Japan, 9%; USA, 19%, Italy, 13%, Brazil, 50%. b) helping people to die painlessly: Japan, 82%; USA, 71%; Italy, 68% and Brazil, 42%. A striking finding in Brazil was that 50% of those interviewed advocated prolonging life for as long as possible. Possibly, this mistaken perception is related to the inadequate use of ICU beds, and justifies the fact that our country is still one of the few in the world that recognizes the use of palliative care in ICUs as justifiable. 2. "When thinking about your own death, what do you consider to be extremely important? a) not leaving your family in financial difficulties: 59% in Japan and 54% in the USA; b) being at peace spiritually: 40% in Brazil; c) having the company of loved ones during the dying process: 34% in Italy. Here, it is worth highlighting the statement "being at peace spiritually", attributed to the vast majority of Brazilians interviewed. 3." On prolonging life as long as possible (data collected only from Brazilian interviewees, taking into account the different levels of education) 51% of those with an elementary education were in favor, while 53% of those with a secondary education had the same opinion and only 35% of those with a higher education welcomed the idea of indiscriminate prolongation of biological life. It can therefore be concluded that Brazilians with a higher level of education favor pain relief and physical and emotional comfort over the alternative of having their biological lives artificially prolonged. (4) Dying with less pain, discomfort and *sufferingAccording* to the other countries studied, 41% of those with an elementary education, 40% of those with a secondary education and 58% of those with a university degree approved of the measure. 5. on who should decide on the medical treatment to be adopted for patients at the end of life: on average across the countries, 57% considered this to be a decision exclusively for patients and their families, while 40% opted for the conduct defined by doctors, and 2% did not know how to respond. In short, the majority of respondents in Japan, Italy and the USA, when dealing with serious and incurable illnesses, chose to receive care that would reduce pain and allow family members to be with them at times close to the end of life, rather than procedures that would artificially prolong life. Furthermore, according to the survey data, 50% of Brazilians, when asked to give their opinion on the end of their own lives, emphatically expressed the wish to remain in an ICU, while in the USA, Italy and Japan, the rates were lower, between 9% and 19% , with the prevalence of the choice for palliative care and a death without pain and suffering. In contrast, in Brazil only 42% considered this option to be "very important". Another finding identified by the survey was the marked prevalence of religiosity among Brazilians, as expressed by the 40% who considered it "extremely important" to be "at peace spiritually" at this time of life's end. Eight out of ten Brazilians (83%) made clear the importance they attach to religious and spiritual convictions. The most noteworthy statistic is when these people declare their wishes regarding the treatment they would like to receive at the end of their lives. In the survey, 54% of Brazilian adults identified themselves as Catholic and three out of ten declared themselves evangelical. The question that arises from the high number of Brazilians who considered the importance of "being spiritually at peace" in the face of imminent death, is how this care is offered. On the other hand, in the USA and Japan, where the cost of medical services is often very high, the condition of preserving the family's financial security after the patient's death is important. In Italy, the greatest concern expressed by patients was that they could count on the presence of "their loved ones by their side" in the final moments of their lives, followed by "the certainty that their personal wishes regarding medical procedures adopted at the end of their lives would be respected". A worrying fact revealed by the research, considering the four countries studied, was the almost systematic lack of dialogue with patients on the subject of the end of life. In Japan, for example, only 31% of adult patients and 33% of those over the age of 65 said they had had the opportunity to discuss the subject with a loved one, and only 7% said they had discussed it with their doctor; only 6% said they had formally made their advance directives, and 64% had not done so, saying they were unaware of this alternative. With similar findings, we point to a study carried out in a private home care service for patients with terminal illnesses in the city of Florianopolis, which was the subject of a Master's Thesis presented to the Master's Program in Bioethics at the Pontificia Universidade Catolica do Parana (PUCPR) in 2016. In the study, the researcher assessed the level of knowledge that 55 patients assisted by the program had about Advance Directives of Will (ADW). Of the total, only one patient had registered their ADW, 3 patients expressed their desire to do so after having had a conversation about the subject with the author of the research, the other 51 patients stated that they had not been given the opportunity to talk about it (SCOTTINI, M.A., 2016). It is well known that the formal registration of VAD is small and varies greatly from parent to parent. With regard to the four countries studied, the results obtained on the subject were as follows: a) considering the general population: 6% in Japan and Italy, 27% in the USA and 14% in Brazil. b) taking into account only the population over 65: 12% in Japan, 5% in Italy, 51% in the USA and 13% in Brazil. Another fact worth reflecting on is the fact that in the USA, approximately 1/3 of people who die after the age of 65 were admitted to an ICU in the months preceding their death and 1/5 of them underwent a surgical procedure in the month preceding their death. It is estimated that by 2020, at least 40% of the US population will die in their own homes or in nursing homes for the elderly, unaccompanied by their families. On the other hand, the chaotic situation of public health services in Brazil, the lack of resources and adequate hospital infrastructure, together with people's insecurity and misinformation, mean that the idea that orthothanasia, i.e. not using futile or disproportionate therapies on patients with incurable diseases in the terminal stage, is considered abandonment of care or omission of medical help, prevails. Mistrust of the quality of the country's public health services favors this misconception. In Brazil, there are 110 palliative care services registered with the National Academy of Palliative Care (ANCP), while in the USA there are 1,700 units. Another huge challenge is the almost total absence of content on end of life and palliative care in the curricula of undergraduate health courses. A study published in The Lancet in November 2010 showed worrying results about the qualifications of graduates from 2420 medical courses around the world. The first pedagogical project used by medical schools at the beginning of the 20th century, after the reforms proposed by the Flexner Report, focused on teaching in tertiary hospitals. The second model, known by its acronym PBL (Problem Based Learning), conceived in the 1970s by the Universities of Maastricht and MacMaster, was widely accepted in health courses. The third model, which promises to train professionals with greater social responsibility, identified as "Health Education Systems", which provides for the training of doctors inspired by the principles of the ethics of otherness, still lacks initiatives for its implementation. The study designed by twenty educators with extensive experience in medical education from different countries around the world, who were part of "The Lancet Commissions", had the main goal of defining the most appropriate professional training profile for practicing medicine in the 21st century (THE LANCET COMMISSIONS, 2010). The proposal to train a new model of professional, better prepared to make reasonable and prudent decisions in the face of the complex ethical conflicts that frequent contemporary society, marked by moral plurality, still occupies the territory of ideals defended by experienced educators, who, however, do not meet the interests defended by university institutions governed by market rules, which prefer to train doctors to serve as many patients as possible, regardless of the quality of the service provided to the community. In this way, unfortunately, we have to recognize that we have not yet reached the goal of training professionals who are prepared to recognize patients as biopsychosocial and spiritual beings, people who have the autonomy to give their opinion and actively participate in the medical procedures that will be carried out on their own bodies. How can we provide professionals with a humanist education when they don't even receive any knowledge about the end of life and palliative care during their undergraduate studies? This is what Pinheiro's study showed when he interviewed 5th and 6th year medical students in the city of Sao Paulo. The survey found that 83% of the students had not received any information on caring for patients with terminal illnesses, 63% had not had any content on "how to give more news", 76% said they did not know the clinical criteria for optimizing pain treatment in cancer patients (PINHEIRO,R.S., 2010). On the other hand, our universities have placed too much emphasis on teaching countless subjects without establishing a logical connection between them that allows students to understand that, no matter what ailment affects a patient, it will always involve the entire biopsychosocial universe of the sick person. The slicing up of the human body into organs and systems that is practiced in most medical schools means that students, and obviously future doctors, are prepared to treat diseases and not people. Edgar Morin is emphatic when he states that "the disciplinary developments of the sciences have not only brought the advantages of the division of labour, but also the drawbacks of overspecialization, confinement and the dismantling of knowledge. They have not only produced knowledge and elucidation, but also ignorance and blindness"

(MORIN, E., 2001). The incipient multidisciplinary approach introduced in medical schools is welcome, but insufficient to deal with the complex moral problems present in end-of-life situations. In relation to human finitude, it is essential that disciplines from different areas of knowledge, such as medicine, psychology, theology, nursing and many others, talk to each other, because only by sharing each area's own knowledge will it be possible to properly care for patients in the terminal phase of life. Only the interdisciplinary approach will offer the means to properly guide the decisions to be made in palliative care (SANTOS, M., 2017). As it seems appropriate, we have recovered the experience of the American neurosurgeon Paul Kalanithi, recorded in his book "The Last Breath of Life", which reproduces the trajectory of his life from the stage "In perfect health I eat" (Part I) to "Not stopping until I die" (Part II). In 167 pages, the author allows us to follow his experience of meeting death. The book's epilogue, written by his wife Lucy after Paul's death, contains the following teaching: *"Paul's decision not to look away from death sums up a strength that we don't celebrate enough in our mortality-averse culture. Writing this book was an opportunity to teach us to face death with integrity"* (KALANITHI, P., 2016). Returning to the research published by The Economist, we consider it important to highlight some points regarding the data found in the four countries studied. Notwithstanding the socio-demographic and cultural differences between them, some points of agreement are worth highlighting, such as the fact that the majority of respondents, regardless of the country studied, considered that health care sponsored by government initiatives was unsatisfactory. A large number of respondents felt that government officials were unprepared or unmotivated to promote appropriate measures for the care of elderly people or those suffering from terminal illnesses. When asked which treatments were considered essential for end-of-life care, the majority of Japanese, Italians and Americans prioritized therapies that would reduce pain and relieve the suffering imposed by the illness. Similarly, when asked about the finiteness of their own lives, there was an expressive consensus: "to live well, as much as possible, as long as the dignity of the person is always respected". When discussing planning for the end of life, the vast majority of people from all four countries said that death is still considered a "taboo subject", which is the biggest obstacle to talking about it. With regard to registering ADRs, North Americans were the ones who showed the highest degree of agreement with signing the document.

8 FINAL CONSIDERATIONS :

We emphasize once again that it is unnecessary to point out the benefits offered to humanity as a result of the technological advances of modern medicine. It is enough to recall the precise information obtained by tomography, magnetic resonance imaging and nuclear medicine, the contributions of ultrasound as a diagnostic method, the decisive value of mammography in the early detection of breast cancer, the detailed information obtained by digestive endoscopy and coronary angiography. From a therapeutic point of view, we can mention the surgeries carried out using videolaparoscopy, microsurgeries and minimally invasive surgical procedures with the help of robotics, conditions that have made the distance between reality and fiction almost non-existent. It is therefore unnecessary to extol the contributions of biomedical technology. However, it is essential to reflect on the appropriate use of all this costly apparatus. We consider it appropriate to recall the lucid statements made by Prof. Jose Paranagua de Santana who, on the occasion of the XXXVIII Brazilian Congress of Medical Education, held in September 2000, said: *"the scientific and technological progress made within the framework of the Flexnerian conception, especially in the second half of the 20th century, is evidence that does not need to be taken into account. On the other hand, and also on this aspect, there is no disagreement, we have observed, rather than stagnation, a frank deterioration in ethical standards in the course of providing medical services"* (SANTANA,J.P., 2000). There is, therefore, broad agreement in condemning the actions that result in the excessively technical and poorly humanistic training of medical professionals. We need to recover the original trust that has always permeated the doctor-patient relationship, because only through this can we understand the sick human being in all their rich and complex dimensions.

In short, the challenge facing us is whether to continue practicing medicine as a technique that is hostage to a growing arsenal of equipment, or to recover perception, reflection and criticism in our professional acts. We mustn't forget, either, that technology is already seducing a huge contingent of patients who very often seek medical care just to fulfill their dream of undergoing the latest procedures invented by technoscience. Confidence in the information provided by equipment is growing in the same proportion as confidence in the doctor's personal competence is decreasing. Will we passively witness the de-characterization of the practice of medicine as an art and accept doctors as docile puppets manipulated by the techno-scientific fundamentalism cunningly sponsored by large medical equipment and pharmaceutical companies?

On the other hand, it is imperative to implement cultural changes that allow us to overcome the topic of death, which is a necessary condition for patients with terminal illnesses to receive adequate palliative care, while being able to count on the physical presence and emotional comfort of their families, as well as spiritual assistance. Only in this way will we recognize them as biopsychosocial and spiritual beings who have the right to die with dignity.

REFERENCES:

BACON, F. *Life and work.* Sao Paulo, Editora Nova Cultura, 1999.

BERLINGUER, G. *Life issues: ethics, science and health.* Sao Paulo: Hucitec, 1993. *Bioetica cotidiana.* Brasilia: Editora UnB, 2004

BIBLE . A.T. Genesis. In *The Jerusalem Bible.* Sao Paulo : Edigoes Paulinas, 1973

BLOOM, A. *The Decline of Western Culture.* Sao Paulo: Best Seller,1989 BOBBIO, M. *O doente imaginado.Sao* Paulo, Bamboo Editorial, 2014

CAIRUS, F.H. RIBEIRO JUNIOR,W. *Hippocratic texts: the patient, the doctor and the disease.* Rio de Janeiro: Fiocruz, 2005.

INTERNATIONAL CENTER FOR TRANSDISCIPLINARY RESEARCH AND STUDIES *What university for tomorrow? In search of a transdisciplinary evolution of the university.* Locarno: Ciret-Unesco, 1997 WORLD COMMISSION ON THE ENVIRONMENT AND DEVELOPMENT. Madrid: Alianza Editorial, 1992.

CORREIO BRAZILIENSE. Brasilia. DF, April 21, 1997 CORTINA, A. *Ciudadanos del Mundo.* Madrid: Alianza Editorial, 2001. ENDO, P. *Sobre a Violencia: Freud, Hannah Arendt e o caso do mdio Galdino.*

In: ZUGUEIB Neto,J.(org.) *Identidade e Crises Sociais na Contemporaneidade.* 'Curitiba: UFPR, 2005.

ENGELHARDT , T. *Fundamentals of Bioethics.* Sao Paulo : Loyola, 1998

ENTRALGO,P.L. *La relation medico-enfermo.* Madrid: Alianza Editorial, 1983.

FREUD, S. *Mas alla del Principio del Placer.* Madrid: Biblioteca Nueva, 1981.

GARRAFA, V. PORTO, D. *Bioetica, poder e injustiga:por uma ética de Intervenão.* In: Bioethics, *Power and Injustice.* Sao Paulo: Loyola, 2003.

GREISCH, J. *De la gnose au Principe Responsabilite: un entretien avec Hans Jonas.* Paris: Esprit, 1991.

HOTTOIS, G. *El paradigma bioetico:una etica para la tecnociencia.* Barcelona: Antthropos, 1991.

HUSSERL, E. *La idea de la fenomenologia:problemas fundamentales de la fenomenologia.* Madrid: Alianza Editorial, 1994.

JONAS, H. *El Principio Responsabilidad: ensayo de una etica para la civilization tecnologica.* Barcelona: Herder, 1995.

KALANITHI, P. *The last breath of life.* Rio de Janeiro : Sextante, 2016 KANH,KL *The use and misuse of upper gastrointestinal endoscopy.* Ann Intern Med, v.109, p. 664-670, 1988.

KANT, I. *Selected Texts.* Petropolis: Vozes, 1985.

LEOPOLDO E SILVA, F. *From philosophical ethics to ethics in health.* In: *Initiation to Bioethics.* Brasilia: CFM, 1998.

LEVINAS, E. *The humanism of the other man.* Petropolis: Vozes, 1993.

LOWN, B. *The lost art of healing.* Sao Paulo: JSN, 1996.

MORIN, E. *El metodo: la naturaleza de la naturaleza.* 3. ed. Madrid: Catedra, 1993. *The well-made head.* Rio de Janeiro : Bertrand Brasil, 2001 MORIN, E. KERN, A.B. *Terra- Patria.* Porto Alegre : Sulina, 1995 NIETZCCHE, F. *A Gaia Ciencia.* Sao Paulo: Companhia das Letras, 2001. NOZICK, R. *Anarchy, State and Utopia.* New York: Basic Books, 1974. PESSOA, F. *Livro do desassossego* .Sao Paulo: Edigao de bolso, 2008. PIKETTY, T. *Capital in the 21st Century.* Rio de Janeiro: Intnnseca, 2014.

PINHEIRO, R.S. *Avaliação do conhecimento sobre cuidados paliativos em estudantes de medicina do quinto e sexto anos.* Mundo da Saude 2010; 34 (3) : 320-26

POPPER, K. *Logic of scientific research.* Sao Paulo: Cultrix, 1972.

POTTER, V. R. *Bioethics;Science of Survival.* Persp Biol Med, v. 14, p.127153,1970.

Bioethics: bridge to the future. New Jersey: Englewood

Cliffs, Prentice Hall, 1971.

Global Bioethics : building on the Leopold legacy. Michigan: East Lansing,Michigan State University Press, 1988

PRIGOGINE, I. *The end of certainties.* Sao Paulo: Unesp, 1996.

CIRET-UNESCO PROJECT *Transdisciplinary Evolution of the University: Which*

*University for tomorrow? In search of a transdisciplinary evolution of the University.*Lugano:UNESCO, 1997.

REVISTA VEJA. Ethics section. February 4, 1998.

SANTANA, J.P. *The paradox of medical education.* Boletim ABEM, v.28, n.4 sep./dec.2000.

SANTOS, M. *Bioethics and Humanization in Oncology.* Brasilia : Elsevier ;2017

SCHRAMM, F. KOTTOW, M. *Principios bioeticos en Salud Publica: limitaciones y propuestas.* Cadernos de Saude Publica, v.1, n.4, 2001 SCOTTINI, M. A. *Advance Directives of Will in patients under home hospitalization at a Medical Cooperative in Florianopolis,* Curitiba. Master's thesis PUCPR ; 2016

SEN, A. *On Ethics and Economics.* Sao Paulo: Companhia das Letras, 1999 *The idea of justice.* Sao Paulo : Companhia das Letras, 2011

SIQUEIRA,J.E. *Etica e tecnociencia:uma abordagem segundo o Principio Responsabilidade de Hans Jonas.* Londrina: UEL, 1998.

. *Ethical reflections on care at the end of life.* Bioetica, v. 13, n.2, p.37-50, 2005.

SONTAG, S. *The disease as metaphor.* Rio de Janeiro: Edigoes Graal, 1984. THE ECONOMIST & LIEN FOUNDATION, *The Quality of death Raakiag end-of-life care access the World ,2010*

THE ECONOMIST &LIEN FOUNDATION , *The Quality of death Raakiag end-of-life care access the World,* 2015

THE ECONOMIST & THE HENRY J. KAISER FAMILY FOUNDATION, *View and Experience with End-of-life medical care in Japan, Italy, The United States and Brazil: A cross-country Survey.* April,2017

THE LANCET COMMISSIONS, 2010 *Health professionals for a new century : transforming education to strengthen health* systems in an interdependent world. The Lancet 2010;6736 (10)

61854-5

TOFFLER, A. *The shock of the future.* Rio de Janeiro: Artenova, 1973.

WEBER, M. *Science and Politics: two vocations.* Sao Paulo: Cultrix, 1980.

______. *Protestant ethics and the spirit of capitalism.* Sao Paulo: Cengage Learning, 2008.

Index

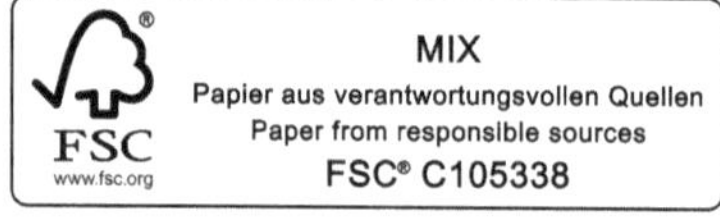

Printed by Books on Demand GmbH, Norderstedt / Germany